WALKING AND DANCING
THREE YEARS OF DANCE IN LONDON
1951 – 53

Larraine Nicholas

The Noverre Press

Photograph on front cover by Eulanda Shead, performed at the University of Roehampton in August 2013 by Georgia Tegou with Stacie Lee Bennett and Dan Worth.

Illustration on back cover, Dancing Britannias: die cut paper souvenir of the Festival of Britain, 1951, designed by Georg Adams-Teltscher. Photo courtesy of Southbank Centre Archive.

First published in 2013 by The Noverre Press,
Southwold House, Isington Road, Binsted, Hampshire, GU34 4PH

ISBN: 978-1-906830-65-6

A CIP catalogue for this title is available from the British Library

Printed in Great Britain

CONTENTS

ACKNOWLEDGEMENTS

As always with research of this kind, I have depended very much on the help and expertise of the professionals in libraries and archives. Kornelia Cepok of the library Archives and Special Collections at the University of Roehampton, where the Monica Collingwood Collection is housed, has been particularly helpful. Staff of the Theatre Museum collections of the Victoria and Albert Museum, where the Lionel Bradley Ballet Bulletins are cared for, have also enabled me to do a considerable amount of the research. Lesley Whitelaw of the Middle Temple Archive generously gave me the benefit of her exceptional knowledge. I also want to thank Emily Churchill of the Southbank Centre Archive who answered some of my questions despite the extreme calls on her time. Sharon Maxwell and Vicky Holmes at the National Resource Centre for Dance, at the University of Surrey helped me access dance journal articles from this period. The preservation values at the NRCD are exemplary. In these times of financial cut backs it is more important than ever to applaud the care and conservation of those very precious ephemera of the past of dance in environments where their value is understood.

My search for moving picture images has been enabled by staff at the Jerome Robbins Dance Division of the New York Public Library and the National Film Archive in London. For still images I especially want to thank Allan Hailstone, whose Flickr photo stream of London, 1949 – 1962 is so evocative of the period, and Ted Loveday, who is busy archiving online the work of his family theatrical design business, Brunskill and Loveday. I have enjoyed corresponding with both of them. Jonathan Gray, editor of *The Dancing Times*, an unsung hero of British dance history, allowed me to access the journal's considerable photographic archives. Eleanor Fitzpatrick of the Royal Academy of Dance opened up the massive archive of G.B.L. Wilson's photographic record of the period. In the complicated world of photographic copyright I have been assisted by some knowledgeable curators and researchers. Greatest thanks go to Biddy Hayward of ArenaPAL who made a lot of enquiries on my behalf. Olivia Stone of V&A Images and Catherine Theakstone of Getty Images have also assisted me as has Alice Standin of New York Public Library. I have researched copyright extensively and if I have breached the rights of any third party I believe I can demonstrate due diligence.

Many thanks are also due to the family of Monica Collingwood. It might have been so easy to dump the collection of her decades of dance spectating as so much rubbish. The fact that they saw its worth is a great credit to them and I have been delighted to correspond with them about details of Monica's life that have made her come alive on the page.

I could not have completed this work without the support of the University of Roehampton. My gratitude goes not only to the University and the Department of Dance in allowing my research leave, but also to individual staff members who encouraged me along the way and covered for me when I was absent (not only physically absent but also absent minded!). My deep appreciation goes to all of you, especially to my colleague, Geraldine Morris, who read my text and helped me to avoid historical and balletic mistakes. Of these mistakes there may still be some, but I claim them all as my own.

Final thanks to David Leonard of Noverre Press/Dance Books and my editor/designer Elizabeth Morrell. Thank you both for your considerable patience and good advice.

Larraine Nicholas, 2013

The Larger Context of Central London Theatres

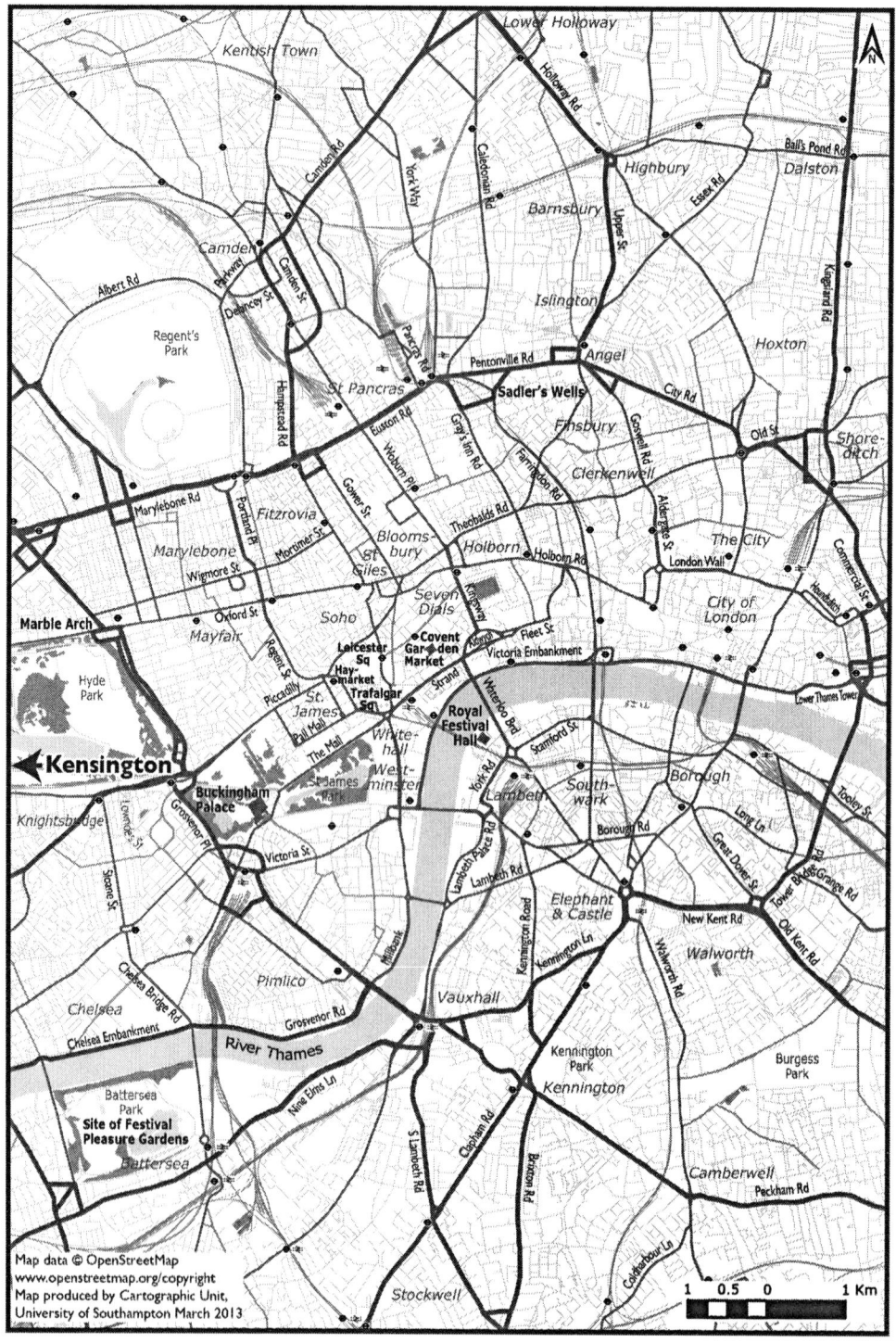

Central London Theatres, 1951-53. Walks and Locations

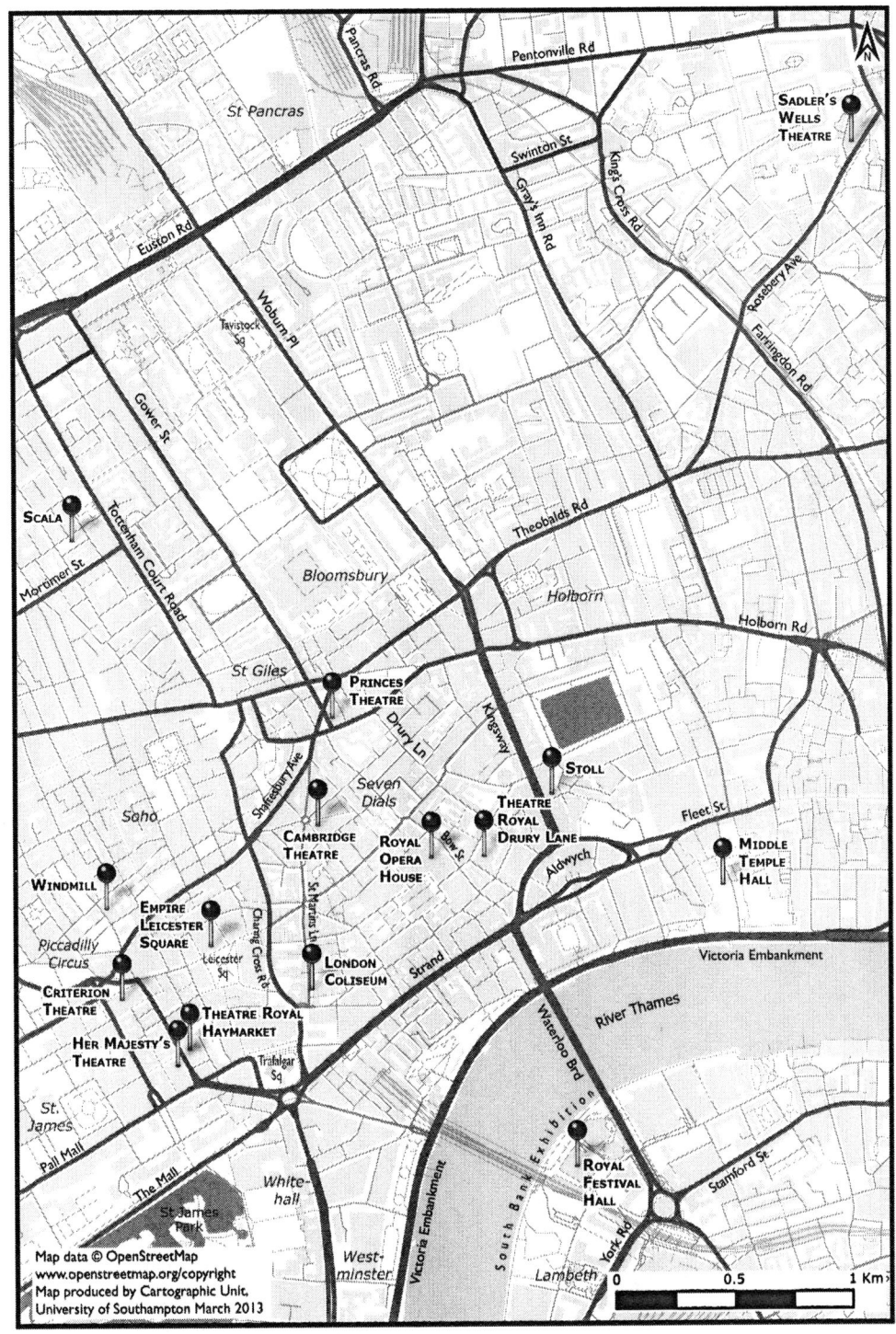

This book is dedicated to all who document and preserve the precious and fleeting moment of dance. The future of dance history is built on the collections of today.

CHAPTER ONE

A (PRE)AMBLE

Sixty years ago

On 4 June 2012 beacons flared on many hilltops of Great Britain. I was one of those clambering to the top of my home village's highest ground where a brazier had just been installed on top of an oak post. In the dusk a herd of cows nosed about with justified curiosity. After an overcast day, the evening was clear and an almost full moon hung over the valley, crossed by occasional wisps of luminous cloud. At ten in the evening our own beacon was lit, followed by others on the opposite horizon, our contribution to the firework displays a volley of sixty rockets, one for every year of the Queen's reign.

Like other official Jubilee celebrations before it, this one was a compromise that conflated the significant dates. Queen Elizabeth II acceded to the throne on 6 February 1952 at the death of her father but the historic point fixed in most minds as marking the new reign is the Coronation of 2 June 1953. The timing of this 60th Jubilee celebration seems to roll these two dates into one, the year of one with the month of the other.

It was the Accession of 1952 that heralded a New Elizabethan Age, to rival the culture, innovation and rising world ascendancy of the first Queen Elizabeth. Apart from the name of the children's magazine, *Young Elizabethans*, the term soon lapsed as the realities of the later 1950s caught up with the fantasy. Tapping the Jubilee moment in 2012, the term 'New Elizabethans' had a temporary revival. BBC Radio 4 instituted a series called *The New Elizabethans*, short programmes profiling sixty Britons who 'defined' the past sixty years in politics, media, culture and sport. Margot Fonteyn was the one personality from the world of dance who made the list. It is worth a comment that sixty years earlier, in 1952, she was also the only dancer on the list of 'New Elizabethans' picked by the magazine *Picture Post*.[1] I discuss the Fonteyn phenomenon later in this book in which I wind a pathway through places and performances of sixty years ago. Fonteyn's reputation is deserved and continued to grow after 1952. However, there is something unsatisfactory in the revelation that the BBC list could not recognise a single other personality representing the growth and diversity of British dance since then.[2]

With the British media in a Jubilee-driven obsession of looking back at the early 1950s and tracing the changes in society over more than half a century, there was a discernible nostalgia. A few days before the Jubilee beacon, I visited a new restaurant, pertinently named 'Union Jacks', opened by Jamie Oliver, the television celebrity chef. The décor was liberal with 1950s style items that in later years became iconic for poor taste, but can now be served up as wistfulness for a more innocent time. We sat at formica tables on a selection of unmatched steel-framed plastic, and wooden chairs, beneath walls decorated by bevel-edged mirrors and rows of those square televisions with the distinctive curved corners of their bulbous screens. Children got special menus to be read with cardboard 3D glasses. Of course the food was not fifties style. Apart from the nod to the gastronomic horrors of the past in the Arctic Roll and Black Forest Gateau on the pudding menu, it foregrounded the local sourcing and sustainability that provide trendy eating in the twenty-first century. But from the national and royal references in its name and the crown on its table napkins, its iconography pointed to a prevailing mood. It seemed that sixty years ago was back in fashion!

Indeed, as the London Olympics of July 2012 approached, the media became obsessed with comparisons with the previous London Olympics of 1948, the so-called 'Austerity Olympics'. As the greyness and hard times of the period, in the immediate aftermath of World War II were mulled over, the implication also emerged that there were some better things then – the people hardier, the life simpler and less acquisitive, the athletes more dedicated to the pure amateur spirit.

The London Olympics Opening Ceremony, *Isles of Wonder*, on 27 July 2012 relayed an often convoluted message. It was truly mammoth in its scope, from Arcadian England, via contemporary popular culture to the invention of the internet. Its opening plumbed nostalgia for the myth of pre-industrial 'deep England',[3] with rolling hills, sheep, geese, yokels, and women in Jane Austen fashions, a perfect land that was disrupted, it seemed, by the industrial revolution. Nevertheless, out of the industrial grime came the symbol of hope, the forging of the Olympic Rings. Children and nurses danced a celebration of the National Health Service, NHS spelt out in the arena in lights. A few commentators sneered, 'It was a social worker's history of Britain, a nation of simple peasants, crushed and besmirched by evil top-hatted capitalists, but rescued in the end by the NHS, immigration, the suffragettes and the egalitarian strains of pop music.' Surely there should be more of the traditional British contributions to the world: Magna Carta, democratic government, the English language?[4] Such critics became entangled in attempting to take a singular narrative from an event so thick with cultural references that many were obscure to foreigners and even to some sections of the British public. Whatever the submerged message, the 'NHS' section was built around a celebration of children's fiction, introduced by a reading from J.M. Barrie's *Peter Pan* and deliberately including staff from Great Ormond Street (Children's) Hospital which became Barrie's legatee. However, it must have been in the minds of the creators[5] that 1948, the year of the last London Olympics, was also the year of vesting of the NHS (the centre-piece of the postwar Welfare State) as well as the year of arrival of the *Empire Windrush*, a ship full of West Indian immigrants (also recreated in the Ceremony).

As a celebration of the symbols of contemporary Britishness, the Opening Ceremony confirmed how many of those are not new, having also been central to the Festival of Britain of 1951 (see Chapter One) – Land, Sea, People, Industry, Innovation. Wrapped up in the symbolism of 2012 was a humour about whimsical juxtapositions, the debunking of pomposity, laughing at ourselves and our treasured institutions – the Queen 'parachuted' into the stadium with James Bond; Mr Bean attempted to play the music and compete in the famous beach running scene of *Chariots of Fire*.[6] This appreciation of the absurd as a trait of British temperament was also present in 1951, in the Lion and Unicorn pavilion of the Festival of Britain.

Dance was also a main feature of the Olympic Opening Ceremony, marking some parallels and some developments over the last sixty years. The prominence of hundreds of amateur performers made an important statement about how community dance for amateurs of all abilities and ages has become an accepted and honourable aspect of British dance. Amateur performance was of course present sixty years ago, in ballroom, folk dance, ballet clubs and Laban guilds. What has changed (at least in some genres) is how that participation is judged, now less by external notions of technical competence and more by the quality of engagement by the participants. The Paralympics Opening Ceremony gave us the performances of professional dancers with disabilities, something that has come into the mainstream only during the past two decades.

Akram Khan's choreography on fifty professional dancers, performed to 'Abide with Me', sung unaccompanied by Emeli Sandé, provided a stunningly beautiful moment of reflection on mortality before the finale of the 2012 Olympic Opening Ceremony. Nothing like Khan's individualistic fusion style of contemporary dance and South Asian kathak could have been seen sixty years ago. Then, London provided appreciative audiences for dancers from the Indian sub-continent such as Ram Gopal and Mrinalini Sarabhai, even though this was before the main immigrations that had brought, amongst others, Khan's parents to Britain. It has been wholly a development of the last half century that contemporary dance aesthetics of American and European legacy have penetrated the dance mainstream. Likewise South Asian dance techniques have become embedded in British dance culture, transcending ethnic boundaries.

British dance performance of sixty years ago was largely centred on ballet technique. When retired Royal Ballet ballerina, Darcey Bussell flew into the arena as the Spirit of the Flame at the 2012 Olympic Closing Ceremony it was a reminder of the continuity of ballet. Sixty years ago British ballet had only just 'come of age', able to compete on international stages. The fame of the British ballerinas of sixty years ago, especially Alicia Markova and Margot Fonteyn, was very potent and they will appear in the following chapters. Despite accusations of elitism and its high financial cost over the past half-century, ballet is still very much with us as a valued and iconic cultural product.

*   *   *   *   *

The nostalgia for six decades ago could be first detected on a major scale in 2011, when the Southbank Centre hosted a season remembering the Festival of Britain and specifically the South Bank Exhibition of 1951. Note how time has closed up the place name from 'South Bank' to 'Southbank'. This signifies a distinction it has taken decades to address: the area around the Royal Festival Hall, on the south bank of the river Thames, is no longer defined as the opposite of the north bank, but now as a cohesive cultural location with a special identity, reclaimed by the city it belongs to. Before 1951, the south bank here was for industries and working-class housing. It was separated from the major cultural and political institutions of London by the river. Then there was the South Bank Exhibition, with the Royal Festival Hall built as the only permanent structure. With the Exhibition subsequently torn up and disposed of, the Festival Hall had to wait until 1967 to be joined by companion venues: The Queen Elizabeth Hall, Purcell Room and Hayward Gallery. But the brutalism of the architecture of the newer buildings and the forbidding concrete of the walkways and stairs made the area hard to love. From 1983, all-day opening of the Royal Festival Hall foyers to members of the public for refreshments and free events began to erode the elitism associated with the concert halls. This policy continued with performances, refreshments and sales kiosks spilling onto outdoor areas. The Southbank became a place for everyone, at any time of the day. Open access festivals including 'Ballroom Blitz' (later just 'Blitz') which from 1990 into the 2000s became a highly significant annual dance event, raised the profile of all types of dance for community participation. After a massive refurbishment of indoor and outdoor spaces between 2005 and 2007 the Southbank re-emerged with a renewed agenda as a place for mass cultural participation.

Visitors to the Southbank Centre in 2011 saw how the spirit of the Festival of Britain and four of its themes – Land, People, Power and Production, Seaside – had been transposed into contemporary settings with twenty-first century values. John Piper's massive mural, *The Englishman's Home*, commissioned for the outside wall of the 1951 'Homes and Gardens' pavilion, was brought back to occupy a whole wall of the Queen Elizabeth Hall foyer (now a lounge, invitingly named Front Room).'Land' came to the urban terraces: roofs, stairways and terraces sprouted gardens, an outdoor installation of wall-building in different kinds of native stone, and a gigantic fox made out of straw sat on the roof of the Hayward Gallery facing Waterloo Bridge, its voluminous brush hanging down the wall, a potent reminder of the collision of city and country. 'Seaside' was enacted on the river frontage, as it was in 1951, now with an urban beach, a giant seagull housing information on seabird conservation, and a row of brightly coloured beach huts, each customised with a display by an artist. 'People of Britain' recognised the inclusion of immigrants and refugees. The voices of refugee children in many languages came from inside a cuboid structure hung with printed poems. This was named The Lion and Unicorn, referring to the pavilion of 1951 that was designed to convey the British character. Back then, it exhibited some of those conventionally held beliefs like democracy and the dominance of the English language, but also a delight in silliness, whimsical humour and unbridled imagination, personified by the unicorn. In 2011 this work of visual and audio art borrowed the symbol of the flying white ceramic doves released by the unicorn in 1951. Now made of paper to match the children's writing, they flew above, taking on new meanings of freedom and hope. The 'Museum of 1951' inside the Royal Festival Hall showed film made for the Festival and original designs and memorabilia. One of its most intriguing exhibits was a living room in what became known as Festival Style, domestic designs that became popular in the 1950s as a result of the Festival: Ercol and G-Plan furniture, wallpapers and fabrics by Lucienne Day, the whole effect was of lightness, busy designs and powerful colour contrasts. Such items are now vintage, collectable and even fashionable (temporarily, no doubt).

The Southbank today has fulfilled the vision of 1951, for 'fun, fantasy and colour'. '[T]his site was never about the few – it was built for the many.'[7] 'Sixty years on the South Bank is beginning to rediscover the Festival spirit.'[8]

The years from 1951 to 1953 included two of the most iconic happenings of the decade: The Festival of Britain, 1951 and the Coronation, 1953. They mediated different versions of Britain which shaped the country's view of itself at mid-century and in some ways set a benchmark for where we have gone since, including the false turns and uncertainties of the twenty-first century. That vexed and contentious pair, modernity and tradition, were balanced differently at different times. In 1951, the predominant story of the Festival was of Britain emerging confidently into the modern world, whereas the symbolism of the Coronation reasserted more forcefully the legacy from the past. The tensions of these years, between innovation and tradition, modernity and heritage, austerity and growth are also current in our celebrations of those events sixty years later. So there is every reason to make those three years the subject of detailed historical research.

A dance history

My historical focus is on London and what it was possible for a dance spectator to view there in the years 1951 to 1953. The variety was tremendous – 'home-grown' ballet companies; musical shows with American choreographers; Spanish, Indian and Indonesian dancers; ballet from America and Europe; variety shows with everything from acrobats to high-kickers and ballet scenes. (This is not an exhaustive list.) The established British dance companies were ballet companies and predominantly used ballet technique since modern dance techniques had not yet made much impression on the mainstream art form. But ballet-trained dancers moved between the established ballet companies and commercial work tracing the outlines of a field of dance activity that embraced film, television, musical theatre and the variety stage as well as the major ballet venues. For British choreographers, ballet was the dominant technique and this dominance is shown in the fact that ballet (iconically, but not exclusively, defined by tutus and *pointe* shoes) was performed in cabaret and in variety, not just on ballet stages like the opera houses of Covent Garden and Sadler's Wells. The versatility of dancers who moved between genres was broadened by the different styles encountered, especially when they came into contact with American-trained dancers and choreographers in musical theatre and variety. This was not new in the 1950s. It was happening pre-war, but the Atlantic crossings were boosted in the postwar period.

By 1951 the institutions of British ballet formed in the 1920s and 1930s had 'come of age', none more significantly than the Sadler's Wells Ballet, under the directorship of Ninette de Valois, made resident in the Royal Opera House from 1946, with a second company in Sadler's Wells Theatre, the Sadler's Wells Theatre Ballet. These were the main focus of Arts Council subsidy on dance. Frederick Ashton was established as the choreographer dominating the Covent Garden stage. The star quality of British ballerina Margot Fonteyn and high profile company tours of North America from 1949 kept these names before members of the public, even the non-ballet-going ones. Occupying this position, on show during grand state occasions at the Opera House, we could suggest that the Sadler's Wells Ballet at the Royal Opera House was evidence of the 'Mandarin values' (aristocratic and reactionary) predominating in public life in the 1950s.[9] This company, and other institutions of ballet at the time, enjoyed the patronage of a royal house dominated, at least in terms of their presence, by women: a dowager queen (Queen Mary), a queen consort (the soon to be widowed Queen Elizabeth the Queen Mother), a female heir apparent (later Queen Elizabeth II) and her only sibling, Princess Margaret.

This picture is a partial one, of course. Other ballet companies toured nationally, some like Ballet Rambert and the short-lived St James Ballet (named after Arts Council headquarters) were publicly subsidised for touring but the largest touring companies – International Ballet, Festival Ballet – were entirely commercial and aimed to be 'popular', that is to attract a non-specialist audience. What is more, this was the age of ballet 'fandom', the 'Ballet Boom', of overnight queues for tickets, when individual ballet stars acquired their own followings replicating film fan behaviour, much to the disgust of some of the cadre of professional dance critics. Ballet in some venues and on some occasions was a perfect expression of 1950s 'Mandarin values' – the place to be seen, formally dressed, in proximity to the rich and the powerful – but at the same time it had its populist side. Dance in the theatre injected colour, movement and escapism into an era of drabness and austerity, but postwar realities also demanded reassessment of the identity of the art form. There were tensions between re-visiting the pre-war repertory and moving on to dance speaking of the second half of the twentieth century. For the ballet stages, many audience members nurtured memories of the Russian and cosmopolitan visiting companies from 1911 onwards, Diaghilev's Ballets Russes and its heirs, and the excitement of London's own ballet pioneering in the inter-war period. How should they move on, acknowledging the past, embodying the present and imagining the future?

The first shake-up came in the late 1940s when London audiences were reunited with Paris, the so recently liberated city. In Les Ballets des Champs Elysées and later with Ballets de Paris, both with the choreographer Roland Petit, London ballet audiences experienced a renewed alignment with ballets that felt youthful, light and chic as well as, controversially, not shrinking from 'sordid' themes, for example the steamy sexuality of the bedroom scene in *Carmen* and a suicide by hanging in *Le Jeune Homme et la Mort*.

British ballet was in the ascendant but challenges to this *status quo* came chiefly from America, echoing the political challenge to world power from the same direction. Soon after the war the Broadway musicals like *Oklahoma!* and *Carousel* (arriving in London in 1947 and 1950 respectively) dominated some of the London stages. Their choreographers used American modern dance idioms which were unfamiliar to British dancers at first. While the slickness and energy were welcomed by audiences, a far cry from the genteel 'musical comedy' style of British musicals, there was some doubt that British dancers could make the transition. Hanya Holm, German/American choreographer of *Kiss Me Kate*, was highly critical: 'Few of them are supple enough, expressive enough. They just don't know how to put dynamic energy into their dancing.'[10]

This challenge was also felt when American ballet companies, American

Ballet Theatre and New York City Ballet, started to visit London after the war. Although even younger than the British ballet institutions, they had clearly set a strongly national stamp on their choreography and performance style. They had Americana pieces such as *Rodeo* (Agnes de Mille) and *Fancy Free* (Jerome Robbins) and shockingly indecorous pieces like Robbins' ballet of sexually predatory insects, *The Cage*. Most unsettling of all was George Balanchine's development of the plotless ballet (*The Four Temperaments* and *Concerto Barocco* for example), choreography stripped to its essential core of dancing and music, sometimes devoid of decorative costume and décor. What should this mean for the repertoires of British companies? Were the nineteenth century classics performed too often to the detriment of new choreography? Was the future to be in new three act narrative ballets or in plotless abstractions *à la* Balanchine? Were revivals of pre-war ballets acts of nostalgia, destined never to live up to the memories? Could British choreographers conceive ballets grittier and more meaningful to the contemporary condition? Would it be possible for musical theatre and variety dancing to emulate American standards?

By 1951, the new world-order had dawned – the Cold War, the division between East and West political blocks, loss of influence and Empire for Britain while American global power was rampant. Some of the emerging factors were not evident on an everyday level. Audiences of the day had no recourse to the hindsight of sixty years later, so in spite of their daily difficulties, there were many signs of optimism. The Festival of Britain and the Coronation reinforced the sense that Britain was still a world power. From the perception of dance audiences and critics, the flourishing interchange between national dance cultures centred on London really gave the lie to any notion that Britain's cultural influence was diminishing. London was repeatedly declared the dance capital of the world. Dance spectators could partake of many dance cultures without leaving the capital.

The narrative of this book closes before the first appearance of the Martha Graham Dance Company in London, in 1954. In hindsight it was a landmark. Coming at the end of the 'ballet-boom', the mainly unreceptive dance public was too challenged or indifferent to its stark language. The prescient few saw that American modern dance could become a major stimulus to British dance but it would take another decade or more to bring these new possibilities into focus, let alone integration into Britain's established dance scene. Catching a whiff of the temper of the times at this juncture of 1953, (I cannot go deeply into it), reveals how unexpected the future can be. Nothing in history is inevitable. My *alter ego*, strolling along the Victoria Embankment on 2 November 1953, has a view of the future of choreography that only partially corresponds with the retrospective view from sixty years in the future.

Walking as methodology and frame

To think historically requires imagination. Knowing sources, evidence and verified data is only a small step towards the leap of understanding that gives even a glimmer of the lives lived in the past. I suggest here that places enable a channel of historical imagination, a structure for making us consider possibilities within a known framework. Places contain within them the potential of their human usage, their human 'dancing in' and 'attending to'. The encounter with places comes through locomotion, of which walking is a basic adult form providing the three-dimensional visual and auditory perspective and also the kinaesthesia of surface texture, light, space and heat. Walking provides maximum capability for stopping, staring, varying speed, varying viewpoint and allowing contemplation. In the real location of past events it has the potential to stimulate thought, imagination and memory. Walking is travelling, and travelling for a purpose is also a powerful kinaesthetic metaphor for reaching a goal or coming to a conclusion.

Travelling to and being in a place of significance seems to be hard wired into us, from pilgrimages, to tourism, to shopping. Historical walking tours abound for any angle on life. We can do walks that reveal the history, geology, ecology, mythology and ghosts of a place. Even dance history can have its walks: the Victoria and Albert Museum published an historical walking tour of London alongside its 2009-2010 Diaghilev Exhibition. It was a journey around the theatres of London associated with Diaghilev's Ballets Russes between 1911 and 1929 (a surprising number of them). This also turned out to be a journey around lost places – the small theatrical suppliers, costumiers and shoemakers needed to get the show on stage but now mainly disappeared from central London.

Walking as a research method, an encounter with the meaning-making inherent between people and places, has had a considerable recent presence in a number of disciplines. Social anthropologist Tim Ingold writes about movement as the fundamental way of achieving knowledge of the world. 'To walk is to journey in the mind.'[11] He acknowledges how city walking is enabled by the technology of footwear and that other technologies (crutches, wheelchairs etc.) also enable this movement which I include in my definition of 'walking'. This layering of the physical onto the mental process is present in real movement pathways but also perceived in visual and audio lines we detect including, music, songs and stories.[12] I add historical narratives to this list.

City walking has its special challenges of traffic and crowds. Michel de Certeau writes of walking the streets of New York as a *Practice of Everyday Life*, like a speech act, with its own rhetoric, based on the enunciation of spatial relationships.[13] It creates its own form of expression, its 'figures of speech' to which he finds analogies in 'the figures of dancing'.[14] I cannot be sure what he means but I would suggest that the modes of locomotion to and from the venue are analogous to these 'figures of speech'. Is it a stroll, a headlong rush, a slog across town, a 'café crawl', a 'walk-and-talk', a balmy or crisp evening on Waterloo Bridge mulling over the performance just seen? Given that we 'journey in the mind' as we approach and leave the venue, there should be some significance in the terrain we tread.

London is also a main centre of the literary genre now referred to as psychogeography, concerned with the strong psychological reaction to place, often revealed through walking. Iain Sinclair, Peter Ackroyd and Will Self are amongst the novelists and commentators who are its current practitioners.[15] My own work is very different to psychogeography, which sometimes veers into the occult, urban ley lines and such. But I take encouragement from their insights about the layering of London's pasts that is evident on the streets, both in the physical environment and in the way it can be presented to imagination. In Chapter One I refer to the writings of Arthur Machen, a London-explorer and writer of a hundred years ago who is much admired by today's psychogeographers.

As I write I want to keep in mind all of this – the analogy between walking the real streets and travelling in thought; stories and histories as forms of travel; the layering of historical topographies on the land that can be reached by imagination; the extraordinary and the intangible revealed through the prosaic act of walking.

Historical narratives need a framing device. Dance histories are frequently framed by a career, a company or genre that is revealed through the ups and downs, climaxes and troughs that unfold over time. In using walking as a framing device I am attempting to realign my selection to the real time of the moment rather than to historical hindsight. This is not to say that I have given up the historian's role in being selective, constructive and critical, but that the walking frame brings new things to light. It has taken me away from the most obvious dance venues to explore interesting juxtapositions of time and place, and performances that acquire a significance they never seemed to have before.

As a dance history, the focus of this book is on some potential experiences of spectatorship within a specific period of dance history. I refer little to the choreographers, their aesthetics and processes. Empirical evidence for individual spectators is rare, other than from the writings of critics so I make no claims for the universalism of the 'we' or the 'I' viewpoints on dance performances in the following chapters. My exploration is rather more into the cultural and political climate of sixty years ago within which dance spectators functioned. Critics rarely situate their artistic life within the socio-political life of the times, but when they do, I take it for evidence that all dance spectators, even those occupying the most remote of aesthetic ivory towers, must notice everyday life, and therefore the match or mismatch between art and life. I aim to present just some possibilities for how it might have felt at performances in London between 1951 and 1953. So this is dance in London as it *could* have been experienced by any anonymous, dance-aware person walking the city, perhaps with a copy of *Ballet* or *The Dancing Times* about their person. However, this hypothetical spectator is not a single person but a conjunction of the twenty-first century researcher, her sources and some diverse, imaginary dance enthusiasts. I hope that my reader can follow me through varying viewpoints and values.

It is essential for my metaphorical journeys through the London of sixty years ago, that there were some dance-obsessed onlookers documenting their experiences. In *The Dancing Times, Ballet, Ballet Today* and *Dance and Dancers*, writers like Clive Barnes, Richard Buckle, Mary Clarke, Arthur Franks, Arnold Haskell, Joan Lawson, Philip Richardson, and Peter Williams documented the dance life of the capital in great detail. Lionel Bradley (1898-1953), a librarian at the London Library, attended many performances as an enthusiast, recording his detailed reactions in Bulletins that he circulated to a select group of other enthusiasts. His persistence in pointing out minor factual errors in Richard Buckle's *Ballet* gave him the chance to write regularly for it.[16] Bradley had an eye for detail, formed by seeing many performances and castings of the same work, making him an expert witness of his time and essential where the dance has been lost to current viewing.

A totally amateur recorder and collector, Monica Collingwood (1913-2003), kept scrapbooks on everything about dance that caught her eye in magazines and newspapers, as well as keeping programmes of just about every performance she ever attended.[17] Enthused at the age of seven by seeing Anna Pavlova, she went on to develop a special attachment to the Sadler's Wells Ballet and Margot Fonteyn, travelling up to London from her home in Coulsdon, Surrey, sometimes twice a week. Her young niece accompanied her on some of these well-remembered occasions.

> There were a whole group of them, ballet nutters! and Monica joined them [in the balcony] when alone, though we always sat in the grand tier whenever I went too. So many memories – the excitement of getting ready, best frocks – ordering the sandwiches for the interval when we got there, handing in the coats to "her special cloakroom lady", an explanation of the story and the meaning behind all the mime moves...it was all pure magic for me as a child.[18]

So the paper trail of discerning observers exists, giving me points of reference for my research. Rarely, though, do they document their journeys as I would like to hear them, embedded in the landscape. Richard Buckle is a notable exception. He loved London, and the sense of London as a real place permeates his prolific writings. Here he describes the walk from Regent's Park to Sadler's Wells for a ballet matinée in the 1930s.

> At a quarter to two at the latest I should have to set off: past Grose's shop in the Euston Road, whose window [was] crammed with the inscrutable paraphernalia of sport... past New St Pancras Church, with an Erechtheion portico tacked on to its side; past the fabulous Gothic hotel where I always wanted to live; past the opening of that long street, with its vista of gasometers, somewhere behind which, entangled in railways, lay little Old St Pancras Church, where Taglioni was married; past the sinister muddle of King's Cross; up the wide majestic Pentonville Road... to the Angel and to Sadler's Wells, 'as to a college situated in a purer air',[19] where keen and chattering queues would be seething and breathing the as yet un-world-famous name of 'Margot'.[20]

In the following chapters walking will enable us to situate performances in real places, arrived at on real London streets of a specific time. Of necessity, imagination being the only means of time travel, my descriptions will have to be filtered through many traces and sources: contemporary accounts, secondary sources and my own observation of dances where possible. In order to strive for a manner of writing that can attempt this unusual project of spectating back in time, the style I use will often diverge from best practice of academic writing. Sometimes the style will be more conversational in order to carry the illusion of a contemporary response and I avoid too much background information on dance works and choreographers. I try to avoid present-day modes of analysis. Endnotes document my primary sources for some of the possible perspectives of the period. I hope that the honesty of this project to get as close as possible to dance of sixty years ago can throw some light on a short but fascinating period that has been given particular significance by the spotlight of sixtieth anniversaries.

The last section of this (pre)amble gives a brief overview of Britain in the postwar decade and of the situation of British dance in the early fifties. These concerns, I would argue, are present in the frame of mind brought to the dance performances by spectators of 1951-1953.

Before we set out, an orientation

On 8 May 1945, V.E. Day marked the end of World War II in Europe. Preparations began in Britain for a general election and the return to normal political conditions after the wartime coalition government. The July election brought about a persuasive Labour Party victory and it was this government which carried through the raft of social legislation creating the Welfare State of which the National Health Service was the central feature. This was not revolutionary in itself, since the postwar reforms were the culmination of planning and reporting which had been ongoing during the war years. In Britain, however, it had a special resonance as a reward for the privations of the 1930s and the war.[21]

During the first three years of the Labour administration, legislation was put into practice which delivered the National Health Service, Child Allowances and a National Insurance scheme against poverty brought about by sickness, age and unemployment. The 1944 Education Act was implemented, raising the school-leaving age to fifteen, and embodying the principle of free secondary education for all. Coloured by the same zeal, but over-optimistic in scale considering the circumstances, a huge building programme was promised to meet the need for new homes, to clear slums and bomb damage. Shocking conditions of insanitary, decaying and overcrowded accommodation in inner cities were still common in 1954 when *Picture Post* published a series of articles, 'The Best and Worst of British Cities'.

The postwar years were to be an era of rebuilding in more than one way. The charter given to the Arts Council in 1946 was also part of this new culture of opportunity for all, now with the notion that enjoying the professional arts of theatre and music was a right for all citizens. Government subsidy of the arts had been a new idea brought about by the perceived need to boost public morale during the war years and ballet companies had become a recognised part of this cultural life. The Council for the Encouragement of Music and the Arts (CEMA) subsidised the Sadler's Wells Ballet, Ballet Rambert and Ballets Jooss.[22] The Arts Council of Great Britain was the direct successor of this wartime role continuing under the chairmanship of the economist and dance-lover Maynard Keynes until his death a few months later.[23] Those ballet companies which had been aided by CEMA continued to be funded by the Arts Council. This was dramatically illustrated by the status accorded to Sadler's Wells Ballet, when it became resident company at the Royal Opera House, Covent Garden, from 1946, acquiring the status of the national ballet company (the charter as the Royal Ballet followed later in 1956). A new company, also associated with the Arts Council, was set up at Sadler's Wells theatre (Sadler's Wells Theatre Ballet), sometimes known as the 'junior' company. Ballet Rambert continued to tour under the direct management of the Arts Council until 1947 when it went on a long tour of Australia, returning to association with the Arts Council in 1949.

The funding of these three dance companies in no way indicates the full extent of indigenous British dance companies in the late 1940s and early 1950s. Just to take the years we are interested in, 1951-53, the major unsubsidised companies were International Ballet (1941-53, dir. Mona Inglesby) and from 1950, Festival Ballet (dir. Anton Dolin).[24] Both these companies feature in the following chapters. A number of smaller companies toured smaller theatres and the provinces.[25] The London dance scene being examined in the following chapters belongs mainly to the large British ballet companies, visiting foreign companies dancing in a variety of techniques, the American musicals with their new choreographic ideas of advancing the story, and the minor venues for variety (but not 'minor' in terms of their popular appeal). Film and television must also be included although the latter, with one channel and not even a complete national coverage, was only just at the beginning of what would become its predominance over other entertainment forms. For most people still in this period, entertainment was a public event.

In spite of all the real achievements of the national postwar settlement, it is clear that, after the first euphoria, there were also reasons for pessimism. The economic effect of the war had been devastating and it was only with the help of an American loan in 1946 and Marshall Aid from the USA (1947-1950) that total bankruptcy was avoided. The late forties and into the fifties have been labelled 'The Age of Austerity'.[26] For one thing, food and clothing continued to be rationed and, under the strain of economic circumstances, rations were cut further, especially after the unusually harsh and long winter of 1946-47. Clothing continued to be rationed until 1949, sweets and sugar until 1953 and rationing finally ended when meat was taken off-ration in 1954. On the one hand rationing was supposed to allow for a reasonably fair distribution of restricted resources, but in reality it meant that somebody, usually 'the housewife', had to spend her time queuing for a commodity that might run out. For those who could afford it, the Black Market was an underhand but also very useful alternative economy. Keeping fed and warm was at the top of the agenda for most people. The Utility scheme had been introduced during the war to manufacture household articles, including clothing and furniture, to reduce waste in the climate of severely reduced imports. These 'no nonsense', undecorated items, were generally of good quality, long outlasting the war and the end of the utility scheme in 1952.[27] However, they retained the connotation of uniformity. Those women who could afford it had already rebelled by adopting 'New Look' fashions with their wide skirts and more extravagant use of cloth after the introduction of the style by Dior in 1947.

Environmental disasters did not stay away either. There were floods with major loss of life. The combination of winter fogs with smoke from the predominant coal used as home fuel created the lethal combination of smog. The early 1950s saw some of the worst of these events, raising London's death rate by thousands. It was not until 1956 that a Clean Air Act was passed by Parliament. There were still bomb sites and uncleared rubble in London and other major cities, terrible reminders of the destruction of the

Blitz. The slow rate of rebuilding homes was for the still homeless a running sore affecting national unity.

Along with the tightening of finances came the narrowing of global influence. The withdrawal from Empire began in 1947 and 1948, when first India and then Burma became independent, and the mandate on Palestine was relinquished. The notion of a British Empire was gradually giving way to one of a Commonwealth of Nations, each self-governing but in most cases still recognising the crowned head of Britain as their own. The formula adopted in the London Declaration of 1949 opened up membership of the Commonwealth (previously confined to the 'white' Dominions such as Canada) to republics such as India. When Queen Elizabeth was crowned in 1953 it was not as empress but as monarch of 'the Peoples of the United Kingdom of Great Britain and Northern Ireland, Canada, Australia, New Zealand, the Union of South Africa, Pakistan and Ceylon, and of your Possessions and the other Territories to any of them belonging or pertaining, according to their respective laws and customs'. The Coronation ceremony resurrected an old symbol of armills (bracelets) of 'sincerity and wisdom'. A gift from the Commonwealth, they stood for a binding force between the Queen and the peoples of the Commonwealth in a new power structure.[28]

Yet none of this could go smoothly. Colonies like Malaya, Cyprus and Kenya had considerable nationalist and anti-colonial insurgencies. In Kenya, the murders committed by the Mau Mau (a cult of Kikuyu tribes) shocked British opinion and the uprising was put down with equal ferocity. Even in nominally independent states such as Iran and Egypt there was strong popular antipathy to perceived occupation based on their unique resources. In the case of Iran it was the Anglo-Iranian Oil Company (later named British Petroleum) leaching off the product with little revenue for Iran. The attempts to nationalise oil assets were defeated in 1953 by a coup in favour of the pro-western Shah, engineered by British and American governments. Those oil crises of the early 1950s have prefigured subsequent crises predicated on the West's reliance on oil production from the Middle East. Egypt still did not have control over its major asset, the Suez Canal, Britain still occupying the Canal Zone. This deeply unpopular occupation was characterised by bloody clashes with Egyptian troops and civilians in the early 1950s, an army coup and declaration of the Egyptian Republic. The Suez Crisis of 1956 put an end to this episode, with a shaming result for Britain.

In the early 1950s the world picture seemed hardly less threatening than during World War II. Atom bombs brought the war with Japan to an end in August 1945 and the prospect of nuclear war came to overshadow all cultural and political activity, with the atom bomb in the possession of both the USA and USSR by 1949, and the hydrogen bomb being tested a few years later. Britain tested its independent nuclear weapon in 1952. This was taking place against the political background of global warfare of a different kind – the Cold War between the ideological blocks of East and West. Its first major conflict was in the Berlin Blockade of 1948-49, when the Soviet authorities controlling East Germany isolated Berlin from land transport necessitating a huge effort to supply the city by air. Then the ideological battle was played out with deadly effect in the Korean War of 1950-1953 between the communist North (supported by the USSR) and the South (supported by the USA). Forces with a UN mandate, including those from Britain and the Commonwealth faced North Korean, Soviet and communist Chinese troops. There was a public fear that this might escalate into nuclear war but the result was a hard-won stalemate and a permanent partition. While on the one hand Britain basked in victory and postwar renewal, the country was still mobilising forces for protection of the residues of Empire, but also for Cold War purposes. Young men continued to be conscripted into the army for two years National Service.

In the austerity and uncertainty of the late forties and early fifties, ballet's illusionism and escapism were attractive. Ballet imagery was appropriated by popular culture, appearing in fabric designs and in advertising, the images accenting lightness, movement and escape from gravity.[29] In 1951, it did not seem strange that the Festival of Britain's logo of the Britannia-headed star could be appropriated to make a paper cut-out souvenir of tutu-ed dancers (see back cover).

This was the age of the 'ballet boom'. By 1949 there were fifty amateur ballet clubs in Britain.[30] This enthusiasm was supported by monthly magazines; during most of the period there were four of them. Leading the field in longevity was *The Dancing Times* (1910 onwards) its great selling power in speaking across the board, to dance public and performers, audiences, social dancers, teachers and learners in all genres. Richard Buckle's journal *Ballet* (1939-1952 with a hiatus during the war)[31], was an idiosyncratic amalgam of the editor's tastes, printing good reproductions of drawings or paintings, not necessarily ballet-related, but also giving space for development of a theme into very long articles commissioned on a variety of genres in dance performance. Two populist magazines emerged in the postwar period. *Ballet Today* (1946-70) was subtitled 'a magazine devoted to ballet everywhere'. *Dance and Dancers* (1950-1994) was edited by Peter Williams, who had previously served an apprenticeship with Richard Buckle on *Ballet*. Both flirted to some extent with being ballet fanzines, showing star photographs on front and back covers; however *Dance and Dancers* pioneered a way of examining new choreography in detail using a number of reviewers. Although articles on ballet predominated, dance in films and musical theatre was also examined. Reading across the four journals condenses a mood of this period, consistently raising questions about the future of dance in Britain. The early 1950s were also characterised by increasing publication of books on dance and successive editions of *The Ballet Annual* summed up each year. Dance stories appeared in popular illustrated magazines such as *Picture Post*. All magazines basked in the glow of London shining out as the centre, as they perceived it, of a global crossroads of dance that included American, Yugoslavian, Danish, French, Indian and Spanish companies.

During the postwar decade the Sadler's Wells Ballet achieved an international reputation, most significantly in America. From 1949, regular winter tours of North America became a feature by either Sadler's Wells Ballet or Sadler's Wells Theatre Ballet, lasting on average twenty weeks, and earning useful dollars. These artistic successes could be given an additional significance within the context of Britain's political situation, as if artistic success in America could compensate for a world political role which had been yielded to the United States of America. Against the background of the Cold War, cultural diplomacy became an important technique for gaining influence within the world political system. The postwar decade presented a world in which there was much to play for politically, but everything to lose if it came to nuclear war. In this atmosphere, with air transport and television making globalisation of culture a simpler proposition, the image of Britain abroad became entwined with the international success of acclaimed cultural products like the Sadler's Wells Ballet .

On 25 October 1951, a month after the closure of the Festival of Britain, a General Election returned a Conservative majority, leaving the government solidly with that party until 1964. The accession of Queen Elizabeth in 1952 and the Coronation of 1953 were moments crystallising expressions of renewed cultural confidence for the country. One of the stories of 1951-1953 is of a nation in recovery but in what way would this be embracing the changed world?

Trials and tribulations at home, dangers from abroad and the comforting certainty of constitutional monarchy are some of the national themes that I see running through the three years, 1951-1953. I keep these in mind for the reader, as for dance spectators of the period, with mini-headlines in the text as events unfold.

Notes

1   'Picture Post Picks the New Elizabethans', *Picture Post*, 19 April 1952, pp.36-43.
2   Fonteyn gave her final performances in 1979. The broadcast in *The New Elizabethans* series on BBC Radio 4 on 10 July 2012 included some astounding inaccuracies.
3   For the term and its significance to national identity, see: Robert Hewison (1995)

Culture and Consensus: England, Art and Politics since 1940, p.23.

4 Peter Hitchens: http://hitchensblog.mailonsunday.co.uk/2012/07/what-sort-of-country-has-a-hospital-bed-as-a-symbol-of-national-pride-and-how-free-is-speech-in-olym/comments/page/3/

5 Film director Danny Boyle and scriptwriter Frank Cottrell Boyce.

6 *Chariots of Fire* (prod. David Puttnam, dir. Hugh Hudson, mus. Vangelis, 1981) was about British runners in the 1924 Paris Olympic Games.

7 Jude Kelly, Artistic Director, Southbank Centre (2011) in *Southbank Centre, Celebrates Festival of Britain, Souvenir Guide* p.1.

8 Barry Turner (2011) *Beacon for Change: how the 1951 Festival of Britain helped to shape a new age*, p.256.

9 For this term see: Robert Hewison (1988) *In Anger: Culture in the Cold War, 1945-60*, revised edition, pp.73-75

10 'Setting Fuse to Dynamite', *Daily Graphic*, 19 January 1951, p.7.

11 Tim Ingold (2011) *Being Alive: Essays on Movement, Knowledge and Description*, p.202.

12 See: Ingold (2007) *Lines: A Brief History*.

13 Michel de Certeau (1984), *The Practice of Everyday Life*, pp.97-98.

14 ibid. p.100.

15 See: Merlin Coverley (2006) *Psychogeography*.

16 Richard Buckle (1953) *The Adventures of a Ballet Critic*, pp.20-23; Bradley's Ballet Bulletins are preserved in the Theatre Museum Collection, Victoria and Albert Museum.

17 Her archive is preserved at the University of Roehampton library, Archives and Special Collections.

18 Communication to author, 14 February 2013.

19 This quotation may refer to the circle of writers who frequented Great Tew in Oxfordshire under the patronage of Viscount Falkland during the reign of Charles I.

20 Richard Buckle (1953) *The Adventures of a Ballet Critic*, pp.66-67.

21 Peter Hennessy (1993) *Never Again: Britain 1945-51*, p.122.

22 Ballets Jooss was a modern dance company directed by an émigré German choreographer Kurt Jooss, based in England 1935-1947.

23 Married to the Russian ballerina Lydia Lopokova, Keynes had a history of interest in the development of British ballet, having been treasurer to the Camargo Society which had produced British ballet performances in London in the early thirties.

24 Continuing under titles: London's Festival Ballet, London Festival Ballet and English National Ballet.

25 For this period the small companies included: Continental Ballet, Ballets Nègres (Afro-Caribbean technique), Ballets Minerva and the British Dance Theatre (modern dance technique).

26 See: Michael Sissons and Philip French eds. (1963) *The Age of Austerity 1945-1951*.

27 I can recall the Utility mark on many items in my 1950s childhood, including bedding and children's clothing. The logo (CC41) was of two black discs with one segment removed like a mouth devouring the number 41 (for the year of the law).

28 King George's Jubilee Trust, *The Coronation of her Majesty Queen Elizabeth II, Approved Souvenir Programme*, pp.30-31.

29 Bevis Hillier (1983) *The Style of the Century: 1900-1980*, p.130.

30 G.B.L. Wilson, (1948) 'Ballet Clubs', in Arnold Haskell ed. *Ballet Annual No. 2*, pp.157-160.

31 Briefly the journal appeared as *Opera and Ballet*, 1948-49, before returning to its former title.

CHAPTER TWO

1951: DANCING BRITANNIA

A Walk to 'the Wells'

When I walk from the Euston Road to Sadler's Wells Theatre, I don't go all along Pentonville Road to the Angel, as Richard Buckle did (see page 12). That would be too noisy and too depressing in 2012. My own route cuts a little way down King's Cross Road and then enters into the quiet Georgian enclave behind Sadler's Wells. I found this for myself but Arthur Machen, one of the elder seers of London's psychogeography, was there before me in the years around 1900. He was an inveterate wanderer without maps, and seeker out of what he titled 'The Ars Magna of London'. The Great Art of London revealed itself to him in moments of almost magical discovery – the effect of a sunset reflected in windows, the view from this hill down into London through the smoky air, the sense that this region was as much *terra incognita* to a Bloomsbury dweller as Africa or the Moon.[1] He had a taste for weird juxtapositions. Walking the streets and squares that were built up in the first half of the nineteenth century as solid middle-class residences, a half century later he found the delectable classicism of Georgian architecture in a living process of decay, as decent terraced dwellings descended into crowded lodgings. He took pleasure in the oddities peeping through the excrescence of the surface – here were also makers of exquisite artificial flowers and other crafts of luxury. The Victorian writer's excitement at the proximity of the underworld is palpable, and in his case it was both the criminal and the occult underworlds that fascinated.

Machen advises me that the Great Art of London, like all art, is a journey into the unknown, so where better to begin a journey into the art of dance but with a factual journey? Of course, what he saw on his walks a hundred years ago and what I see now are quite different in some respects. Now the cycle of gentrification has made these desirable addresses and some have returned to single family ownership.[2] Although the area is still quiet in contrast to Pentonville Road or Rosebery Avenue, unfortunately I cannot confirm Machen's observation that a car, a taxi or bus is never seen here. But this is still the 'green grove' he describes. 'For trees grow everywhere in this happy place. They lean over garden walls, they congregate together in hushed squares, they swell richly from little patches of odd ground, from behind railings, in every unexpected quarter'.[3] Unlike Machen, I don't wander for the sake of it but in order to reach Sadler's Wells. My walk gives a clue to the historical meaning of the theatre – it's all about air and water!

Imagine standing on the hills of northern Clerkenwell (now Finsbury and Pentonville) in the seventeenth and eighteenth centuries, feeling the spacious countryside after the squalid city and enjoying views down into smoky London. And then, imagine that you have a mind for entertainment. 'Wells' and 'Spas' abound here, one of them leased to Edward Sadler in 1671 and ever after retaining his name.[4] If the medicinal waters lack current attraction, there is plenty of alcohol on offer along with performances that don't demand too much cerebration. As for the water, the natural supply is superseded in volume and influence by the man-made supply of the New River, bringing drinking water to London. It's not a river but a channel cut from villages in Hertfordshire. (Chadwell and Amwell are village springs that give their names to streets on my journey to Sadler's Wells). The course of the New River runs by Sadler's Wells along what will become the future Rosebery Avenue in 1892, pooling finally at the reservoir of New River Head, Sadler's Wells's immediate neighbour on the South West.

Moving further forward in time to the first half of the nineteenth century, the period when the fields around are being developed for housing, Sadler's Wells is now a spectacular venue, much improved inside and outside. The entrance is in St John's Street, east of where it is now, and the New River makes a promenade on the south of the theatre, lined by railings and trees. In the background is the Round Pool or reservoir of the New River Head. The theatre gives water dramas, a huge stage tank filled from the New River and later even a waterfall. Here we can see fireworks, sea monsters and naval battles as well as plays and pantomimes with the famous clown Joseph Grimaldi. As a major landlord of this area, the New River Company is mainly responsible (along with the Lloyd Baker Estate) for building the residential streets of my walk to Sadler's Wells, always having to invent designs to avoid their own water mains supplying the city. On all levels, the presence of water structures the land and its use. In the 1860s, with the majority of the residential properties built up, the New River is buried and the Wells subsequently gets a new entrance on what will become Rosebery Avenue. The ups and downs, extensions and rebuildings, of the next half century culminate in what seems to be final closure in 1915 and dereliction. The story of the theatre's recall to life in 1930-31 by Lilian Baylis of the Old Vic is well known. The rebuilt theatre, opened in 1931, becomes central to the development of Ninette de Valois' Vic-Wells Ballet, later named Sadler's Wells Ballet. Joseph Hermon Cawthra's frieze above the Rosebery Avenue entrance depicts women drawing water from a well, confirming again the watery connections of Sadler's Wells.[5]

Changing voice, I'm now a walker from King's Cross Road to Sadler's Wells in 1951 (not Arthur Machen as he died away from London in 1947.) I admire and am pleased to see how much war damage has already been repaired although building work for the social housing project to replace the

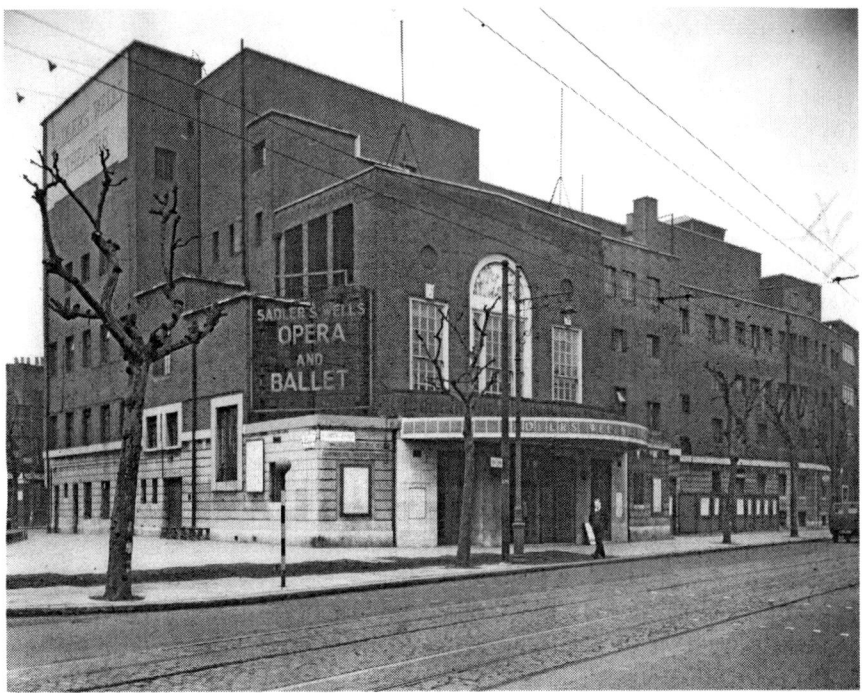

Sadler's Wells Theatre from Rosebery Avenue in 1951. Photo: © Topfoto/ ArenaPAL.

bombed-out Holford Square with the modern flats of Bevin Court (named after Labour Party minister Ernest Bevin) is still very evident.[6] The New River has been halted at Stoke Newington since 1946. The sites of the ponds and filter beds are obscured from view behind the walls of the Metropolitan Water Board. Still 'the Wells' is in all our minds a place for air and water. We ballet enthusiasts go there to see the 'junior' company, Sadler's Wells Theatre Ballet, but no longer Margot Fonteyn, since she is now star of the ballet at Covent Garden. We crowd into the tiny foyer or take the side entrance to the gallery where we chatter with the other regulars. We occasionally see *Swan Lake* (Act II, the Lakeside) and reflect perhaps, that water is always appropriate at 'the Wells'.

February 1951
8th : Elections in Gold Coast [later Ghana] give victory to Convention People's Party (leader Kwame Nkrumah), calling for speedy move to independence from Britain.

March
14th : In South Korea, Seoul is recaptured from communist forces by UN troops.
15th : Iranian parliament nationalises Anglo-Iranian Oil Company at Abadan.

In 1951 alone Monica Collingwood attends 55 dance performances! She is devoted to the Sadler's Wells Ballet, adores Margot Fonteyn, tries to see every one of her performances and makes her the exclusive subject of some of her scrapbooks. Monica is an ardent follower of the repertory, old and new, and of various castings. On 21 February the Sadler's Wells Ballet performs back at the Royal Opera House for the first time after its triumphant North American tour. This is also the fifth anniversary of the company's opening at its new home here. As then, the ballet is *The Sleeping Beauty* with Margot Fonteyn. Lionel Bradley writes that she 'has come to a degree of perfection which entitles her to be considered, apart from Danilova and Markova, the greatest classical dancer outside Russia'.[7] Though Monica apparently misses this occasion, she once more becomes a regular at the Opera House. In March she sees fifteen performances here and at Sadler's Wells. At the Royal Opera House she watches Fonteyn ('Wonderful!')[8] and Michael Somes in *Sleeping Beauty* four times, three times in *Cinderella*, and once in *Swan Lake* ('Lovely'); allowing herself just one alternative casting in *Sleeping Beauty* of Violetta Elvin and John Hart, and of Elvin and John Field in *Swan Lake*.

Monica's tally is only half of the amount Lionel Bradley chalks up in his semi-professional capacity. He reports on one hundred and ten productions in his Ballet Bulletins for 1951, including operas with dancing. His tastes are more eclectic than Monica's. As well as ballet at Covent Garden and Sadler's Wells, he strongly supports Festival Ballet, the new company headed by Alicia Markova and Anton Dolin and all the visiting companies. He maintains a special regard for Ballet Rambert, attending their occasional seasons at the King's Theatre, Hammersmith, at the very margins of London. On Sundays he attends Ballet Workshop, the platform for new choreography that has just been instituted at the tiny Mercury Theatre in Kensington (the origin and homeland of the Rambert organisation).

Up at Sadler's Wells on 13 March Monica sees the premiere of *Pineapple Poll* on a programme devoted to its choreographer, the rising star John Cranko, though it is his *Beauty and the Beast* that she notes is 'beautiful'. She sees *Beauty* and *Poll* twice again in March on different programmes. What does she think of *Pineapple Poll*? Scrutinising the reviews for likely pieces for her scrapbook she may notice these.

> [T]he national flavour is so inherent throughout that the Festival of Britain will be hard put to it to produce a more topical, more praiseworthy offering.[9]

Or:

> The ballet is absolutely English in essence, for Cranko has brought out all the salient points of our comedy traditions.[10]

Monica will understand what this means. In March, ahead of the Festival that is due to take place from May to September, everybody knows that the country has been promised 'fun, fantasy, and colour', controversial as this is

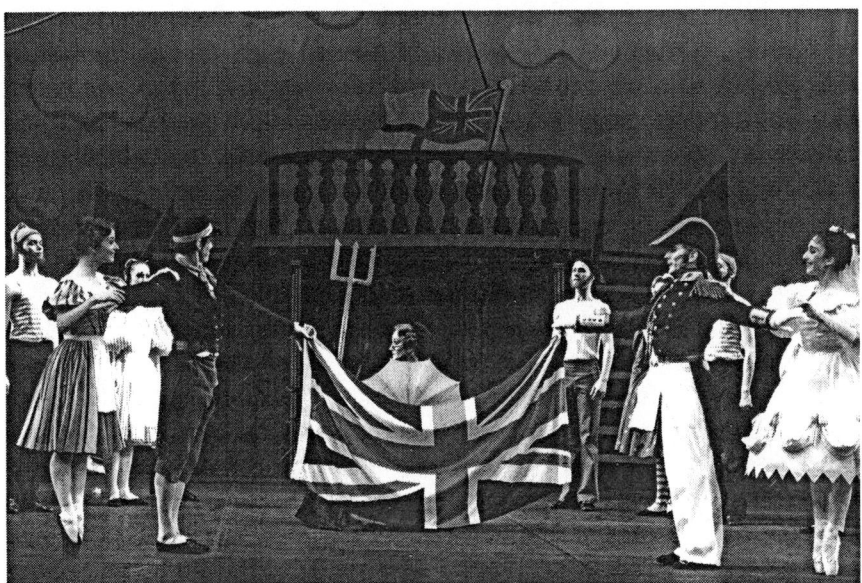

The finale of *Pineapple Poll* (chor. Cranko, 1951) where Mrs Dimple becomes Britannia, from a Birmingham Royal Ballet production, 1995. From left: Poll (Sandra Madgwick), Jasper (unidentified), Mrs Dimple (Chenca Williams) Captain Belaye (Michael O'Hare) and Blanche (Simone Clarke). Photo: ©Angela Taylor.

at such a moment of austerity. The Festival of Britain is to hold up a mirror to the people, showing British attributes and values, when:

> we can, while soberly surveying our great past and our promising future, for once let ourselves go, and in which the myth that we take our pleasures sadly will finally be disproved.[11]

The *Pineapple Poll* that Monica sees is loosely based upon a *Bab Ballad* of W.S. Gilbert with a score arranged from music of the Gilbert and Sullivan operas[12]. It is a typically Gilbertian story of love, initially unrequited; of characters drawn boldly for their vanity, pathos and comic potential; and of romping good humour. Its setting, designed by cartoonist of *The Daily Express*, and observer of class-based absurdities, Osbert Lancaster,[13] is themed as both Victorian and nautical: these are defining institutions of British identity, subjects of justifiable pride. Poll, like all the women of Portsmouth – 'Sweethearts, Wives, etc.'[14] – is in love with the handsome Captain Belaye. In turn, she is loved by Jasper, a common and awkward cleaner-up (pot boy) at a local inn. While women swoon around him, Belaye dances (hornpipe steps, naturally!) conceitedly aware only of his own faultless technical ability, in skippering as in dancing.

Poll and the other women disguise themselves in sailors' uniforms to be near the object of their devotion aboard his ship, HMS Hot Cross Bun. The rigours of the man o' war (cannons, drill, orders!) test their nerves.

Finally, much more to their distress, they learn that he has become engaged to Blanche, a vacuous girl he clearly adores, even though constantly distracted by a dreadful chaperone, Mrs Dimple, chattering incessantly and dropping her belongings. When the men of Portsmouth burst on board, the women are quite ready to accept their disappointment, beg to be forgiven and reunited. Poll warms to Jasper seeing how good he looks in the naval captain's uniform he is given (for no clear reason). The final tableau elevates Mrs Dimple. Draped in the union flag and with her umbrella as a shield, she becomes the whimsical personification of Britannia![15]

In March 1951 the topicality of the ballet is in its innocent allusions to the glories of the Victorian period: Gilbert and Sullivan, Empire and Royal Navy (the 'Senior Service', also a brand of cigarette), presided over by the helmeted and steadfast figure of Britannia, the symbol of national unification, familiar from the back of the one penny coin in everyone's pockets. To a winning but exhausted nation from the recent war, these are all symbols of comforting stability. On posters and advertisements, Britannia's head surmounting a four-point star is now becoming the distinctive emblem of the Festival of Britain.[16] Yet the ballet wraps up its pride in self-deprecating comedy. With its lovelorn women dressed up as men, jaunty sailors and scatter-brained chaperone, the stock characters of *Pineapple Poll* would be at home, not only in a Gilbert and Sullivan opera, but also in the music hall and pantomime. It is a supposed tradition that Britons are capable of laughing at the institutions they hold most dear.[17] One critic quips that 'Lord Festival' (i.e. Herbert Morrison) could justifiably commandeer *Pineapple Poll* and run it as a Festival of Britain attraction.[18] Bradley simply records that, if he could see *Pineapple Poll* every day, it would be all the tonic he needed.[19] If we want any further evidence of how the ballet and the national moment speak to each other, we can buy that simple Festival of Britain souvenir of cut-out dolls, each one a *tutu*-ed and *pointe*-dancing Britannia based on the Festival Star (back cover). Nationalism is combined with brightness and levity.

April

11th : The Stone of Scone, stolen by Scottish nationalist from Westminster Abbey, is discovered in Arbroath Abbey and returned to the Coronation Chair at Westminster.

May 1951

3rd : The Festival of Britain is opened by King George VI and Queen Elizabeth with a service at St. Paul's Cathedral, a guided tour of the South Bank Exhibition and an evening concert in the Royal Festival Hall.
11th – 28th : After numerous delays, opening in stages of the Festival Pleasure Gardens at Battersea.
12th : USA tests hydrogen bomb.

June

7th: Because of the King's ill-health, Princess Elizabeth, on horseback, takes the salute at Trooping the Colour to celebrate the King's official birthday. King Haakon of Norway watches the ceremony and afterwards visits the South Bank Exhibition.

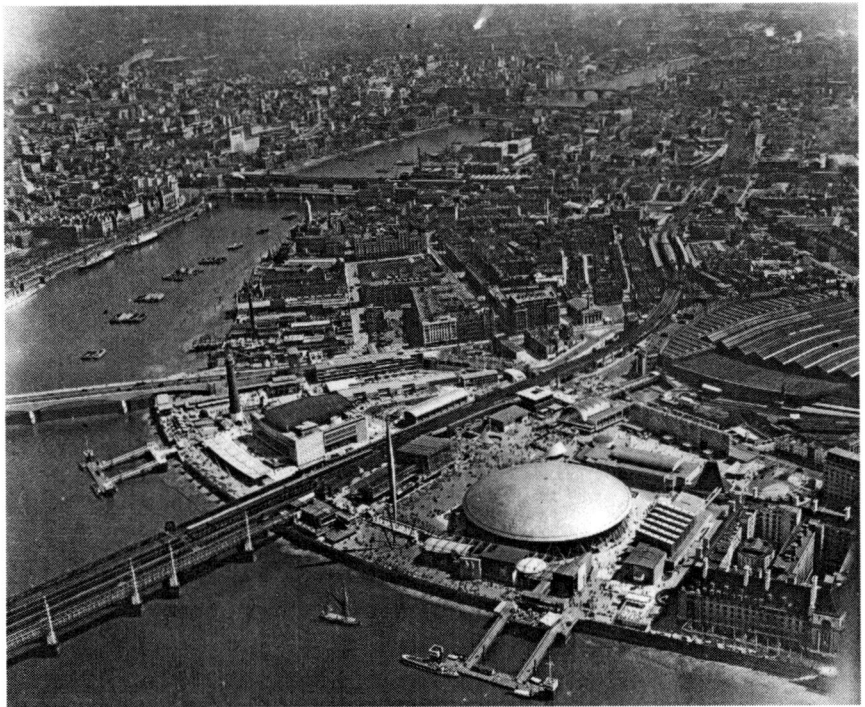

Aerial view of the South Bank during the Festival of Britain, 1951. Major structures along the River from the right: County Hall, the Dome of Discovery, Skylon, Hungerford Bridge, Royal Festival Hall, Shot Tower, Waterloo Bridge. Photo: © Central Press/Getty Images.

To the South Bank

While the Festival achieves a countrywide spread, it is the Festival in London where we are to walk, and particularly beside the Thames. Science, architecture, books, films and the arts all have their place in the Festival season around the capital but on the Thames two major undertakings are soaking up the money: the South Bank Exhibition near Waterloo Station and The Festival Pleasure Gardens at Battersea.

The South Bank Exhibition is a complex of pavilions, urban landscaping and public art, tightly storyboarded to deliver a grand narrative of nationhood, 'The Autobiography of a Nation'.[20] Prominent in all the exhibits is the official 'Way to Go Round'. So keen are the curators on the narrative of the exhibition, that mere wandering is discouraged. Soon after the Exhibition closes, almost the only building remaining will be the Royal Festival Hall, a new major concert hall which will provide a new venue for dance. Another will be the Telekinema (quite soon Telecinema is more acceptable as a contemporary spelling) where film and television programmes, some in 3D, offer other prospects for entertainment. The

Exhibition itself is powerfully scripted, rhetorically educational in manner, arranged in two circuits, upstream and downstream of Hungerford Bridge over which trains rattle between Charing Cross and Waterloo. The Upstream Circuit tells the story of the Land of Britain, and what the people have derived from it, including its resources, products and industries. Praising British ingenuity and labour, here also is the Dome of Discovery (land, sea, polar ice caps, and space) and the vertical structure, the Skylon. The Downstream Circuit, grouped around the Royal Festival Hall, tells the story of the peoples of the British Isles and what the land had made of them. Here is the Britain of postwar reform and the welfare state ('The New Schools', and 'Health'); domesticity and pastimes ('Homes and Gardens', 'Sport', 'The Seaside'). Here also is the celebration of the British temperament, the quirky 'Lion and Unicorn' pavilion. Not only does it celebrate obvious matters of national pride – the English language, Shakespeare, the Church, democracy – but also eccentricity and imagination, those qualities symbolised by the unicorn and illustrated by life-sized characters from Lewis Carroll and crazy inventions, such as a 'smoke grinding machine'.[21]

It seems incredible that, up to three years before this, it was a dismal area of wharves, factories and terraced houses, and a disused brewery. The only building retained for the exhibition is the tower for manufacturing lead shot, now converted with a beacon at its tip to demonstrate radar. Never before counted as a flower of the capital's culture, the South Bank now becomes synonymous with modern design and a colourful optimistic future. The architecture shows clean, uncluttered lines. Science offers symbolism for design, in the atom and molecule motifs everywhere.

The Festival Pleasure Gardens at Battersea have quite a different aura. If 'fun, fantasy and colour' are to be expected in the Festival, this place is full of it. The invocation from the Official Guide Book greets visitors in 1951 with a long poem concluding:

Think what you will. We hoist the Flag of Fun
We bid you
WELCOME
—and we pray for sun.[22]

The tour I now propose is one of imagination in which the guide book mapping of the Battersea site combines with primary sources. It is June 1951. Why are we here? Paradoxically this is where the regular dance performances of the South Bank are to be found, not in the Royal Festival Hall, not yet anyway.

We can land by boat from the South Bank Exhibition downstream, or walk through any of the land-side gates. The Gardens are laid out for strolling,

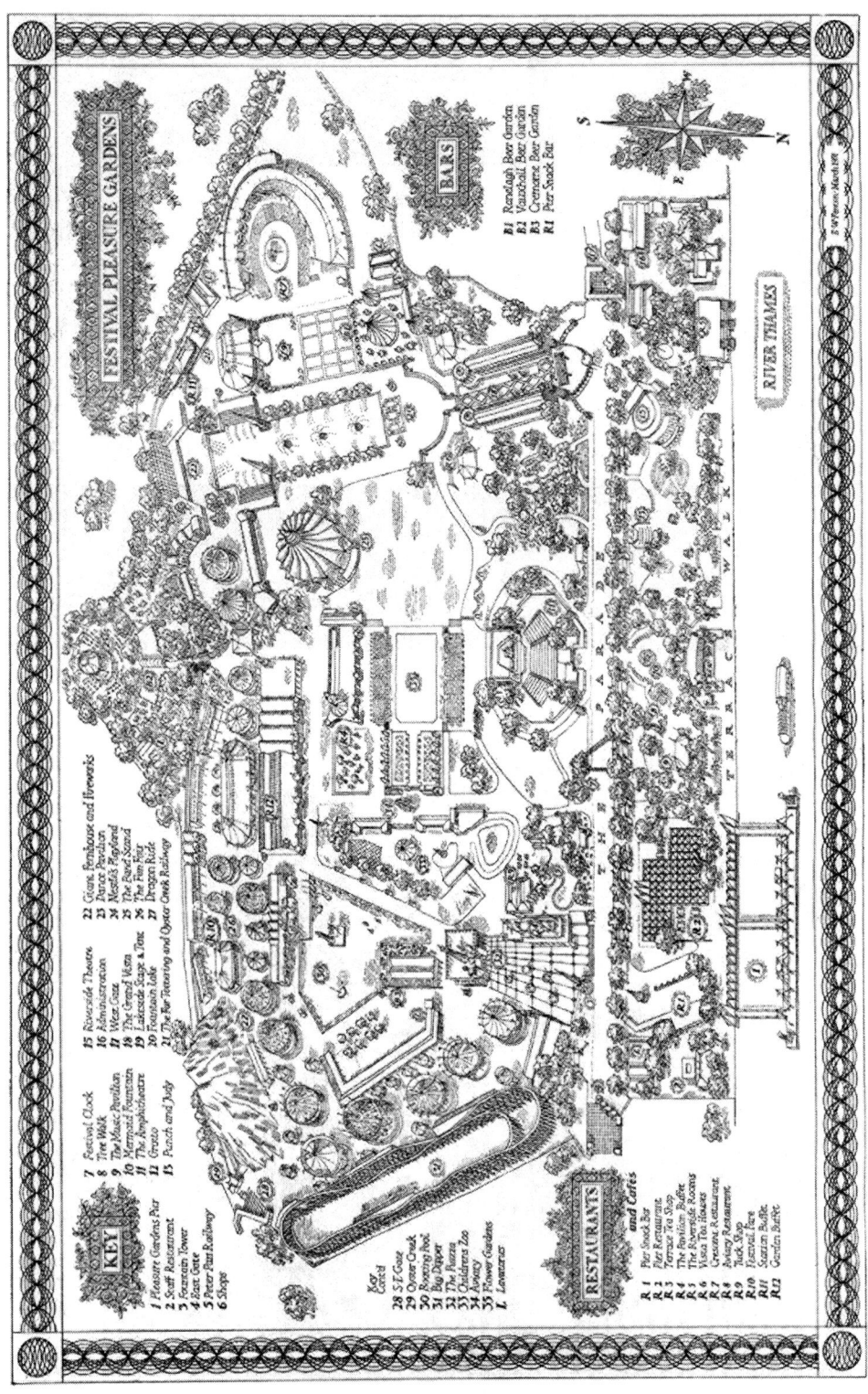

Plan of the Festival Pleasure Gardens, Battersea, from the Official Guide, 1951. Amphitheatre (no. 11), Riverside Theatre (no. 15), Dance Pavilion (no.23).

unlike the definitive 'Way to Go Round' of the South Bank Exhibition. The Riverside Terrace and The Parade run parallel to the river, and a continuous route round the edge of the site allows ways through to the extraordinary features that catch the eye. There are big set-piece constructions. The Grand Vista by John Piper and Osbert Lancaster has lakes and pyramidal fountains, stretching in the distance to the Fern House, a tracery structure like the Crystal Palace of 1851.[23] The Far Tottering and Oyster Creek Railway (the 'engineered' version of what started as a cartoon by Rowland Emmett) travels to the Funfair, and the Big Dipper. Up a spiral staircase, the tree walk is an over-ground path, suspended amongst trees and passing back and forth over the people strolling along The Parade below. Here is a village of houses and shops called Branchville, a swinging cat, and huge dragon flying alongside the walkway. At the entrance tower, automated figures constantly move in and out, looking at the sky ('we pray for sun', indeed!) and at the exit, metal birds are released from a cage.

While the South Bank Exhibition takes design features from technology (crystals, atomic structures, futuristic shapes) and modernist architecture, the Pleasure Gardens opt for fantasy landscapes, with multiple historical references. We see baroque piazzas, a Mississippi showboat, medieval tents with fringes and pelmets; the pleasure gardens of eighteenth century London; coloured canvas from traditional fairgrounds; castle towers, arches, cupolas and Gaudiesque spires. It is truly a sensuous experience. Colour is a continued theme. The Dance Pavilion (currently the largest single pole tent in the world) is of scalloped yellow and brown fabric with a red carpet. Blues, whites and gold abound: the white and gold extravaganza of the Pavilion Buffet, the succession of annual flowers, the Wedgewood Blue of the Riverside Theatre. Strolling along the Riverside there is music gently pumped through loudspeakers. These are records (78 r.p.m. no doubt!) placed onto turntables by a real person in the HMV Music Pavilion. In the Grotto (sponsored by drinks manufacture, Schweppes), there are caves for Wind, Fire, Earth and Water climaxing in the Temple of the Winds. Each wind has its own smell and sound – pines and sleigh bells from the North, spices and temple bells from the East.[24] The Guinness clock chimes out every quarter hour with automata, including the famous Guinness pelican. Children shout at the Punch and Judy Theatre and at the Lakeside where there are acrobats and aerial acts.

The Gardens at night are lit by lamps like birdcages or flowers, the traceries of branches outlined by fairy lights and the houses of Branchville showing lights in their windows. A lighthouse illuminates the boating pool. Chandeliers hang over the Grand Vista and the pyramidal fountains glow from inside. And there are fireworks! Imagine this in a city that has so recently been plunged in blackout.

Now to look for dancing

The Dance Pavilion, that huge tent of yellow and brown, is open from 3pm until 11pm. Admission to the promenade is free but dance tickets cost sixpence. An eyewitness gives an opinion.

> We first struggle through the crowds of spectators, who outnumber the dancers by about eight to one, to find the right queue for the purchase of a dance floor ticket. Another struggle to get into the right queue for the dance floor, and in a little while we are actually on the dance floor, a magnificent new maple one, far too good for the job. We deposit our hats, coats and handbags in a heap at the foot of the main mast of the tent ... we dance for a little while, the music stops, we collect [them].

Most people do not dance, pay nothing, just watch and listen to the barely adequate band. What is more, the dancing is not serious, according to this reporter, as *ad hoc* and silly as the fairground attractions next door. Why not let people dance for nothing since it doesn't seem to be making any money?[25] Is it concern for finance, shyness, or lack of interest that stops people from joining in? I would rather be free to wander in and out at will. This is where the stroll is better than the guided tour! The movement and music mixing with the other fairground sounds, and the 'trick lighting, rather like a gigantic bunch of illuminated leeks', are totally in keeping with the other sensuous delights of the Gardens.

The open air Amphitheatre has rows of banked seating with a stage at the far end. A half-hour ballet is performed twice a day, at 6.30 pm and 9.00 pm. *Orlando's Silver Wedding*, is based on Katherine Hale's children's books about Orlando the Marmalade cat with music by Arthur Benjamin ('quite pleasant and cat-like' says Lionel Bradley), incorporating songs that tell the story. Orlando is abducted by the Katnapper and must be rescued before the Silver Wedding party can be celebrated. Meanwhile, his wife Grace is assailed by four suitor cats who are scared off by the three kittens, Pansy, Blanche and Tinkle. Other feline characters include a Siamese Can-Can Cat, a Blue Persian and different kinds of tabby. Any reasonable ballet fan coming to the Amphitheatre realises that this is not an amateurish production. Its balletic credentials are impeccable, choreographed by Andrée Howard, whose previous works have been in the repertory of Ballet Rambert and Sadler's Wells Theatre Ballet.[26] The dancers are first rate. Harold Turner as Orlando, has danced for Rambert, Vic-Wells (Sadler's Wells) Ballet and International Ballet. Grace is Sally Gilmour, previously ballerina with Ballet Rambert and now, more importantly, she has relinquished her star dancing role as Louise in *Carousel*, across the river at Drury Lane Theatre, in order to perform here! Other dancers in the cast are well known in ballet and/or musical theatre performances.[27] The décor is all scaled up to make the 'cats' look their proper

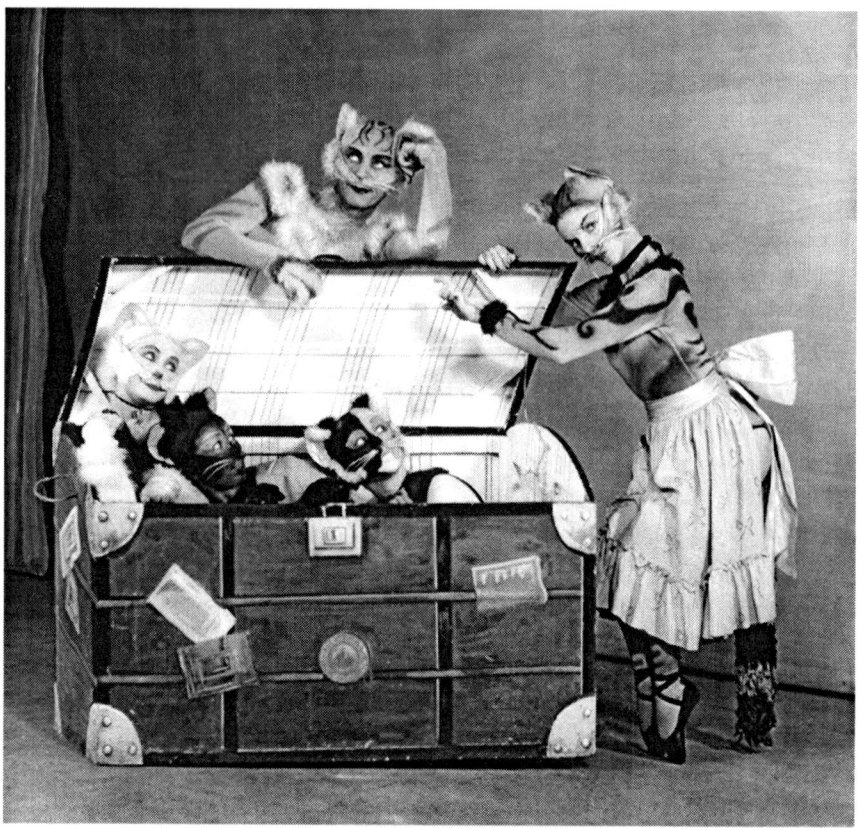

Harold Turner as Orlando and Sally Gilmour as Grace in *Orlando's Silver Wedding*, 1951. The Kittens are performed by Joy Carter, June Leighton and Grace Greenaway. Photo: © Gordon Anthony/Getty Images.

size, including a huge telephone and the tricycle on which Grace races to save Orlando. As with the Dance Pavilion, few people pay to sit down in the two shilling or one shilling seats. They can stand at the back for nothing if they like, and many do.[28] Come across almost by accident, here is a live performance of music, song and dance, short in duration but expertly fitted to the spirit of the Gardens. Lionel Bradley considers it 'small beer but it is charmingly presented and very well danced.'[29] After *Orlando* comes a popular variety programme, The Lambeth Walkers hosted by Lupino Lane. The simple conceit is that it all happens in a cockney pub with acts including 'that amazingly gifted long-legged' dancer, Kim Kendall.[30]

A rather different venue is the blue Riverside Theatre. It has proper, tip-up plush seats for around 400 paying audience in stalls, circle and gallery. The circle is scalloped to resemble boxes, with a promenade to the rear. This intimate little gem is decorated inside to imitate a miniature old-time music hall, with swags, tassels and chandeliers. The painting on ceilings and surfaces imitates the stucco ornaments and gilding of 'proper' theatres of the age. It's a temporary building but made to be taken down and reconstructed.[31]

Of the performances here, we might find the regular 'Seven O'Clock Show' particularly interesting in early June. Liong, Tamara and Edo Sie perform a programme of 'Traditional Balinese Dances'. Lionel Bradley records that it's a 45 minute programme of four dances with an interval in which a pianist plays French music. Tamara performs solos, a girl making offerings to a goddess and a haughty queen at her *toilette*, while the brothers accompany her on *gender* (a gamelan instrument) and drums. Then the brothers perform dramatic dances with accompaniment from their sister. In *Baris Kembar* they interpret the story of twin brothers resorting to murder over who should succeed their father as king and, in *Tjalonarang*, Liong as Prince Pandun kills Rangda, Queen and mother of witches, Edo in this role letting out some bloodcurdling yells that quite impress Bradley.[32]

Then at 10 pm on the same stage is the nightly 'Mr Sachs's Song Saloon'. These 'Scintillating Varieties' are an outpost of the popular 'Victorian' music hall at the Player's Theatre, under the railway arches near Charing Cross Station. Leonard Sachs is the master of ceremonies, with a gavel and hyperbolic phraseology, leading the sing-along and introducing the acts.[33] Amongst the songs and sketches are to be found what he would no doubt call

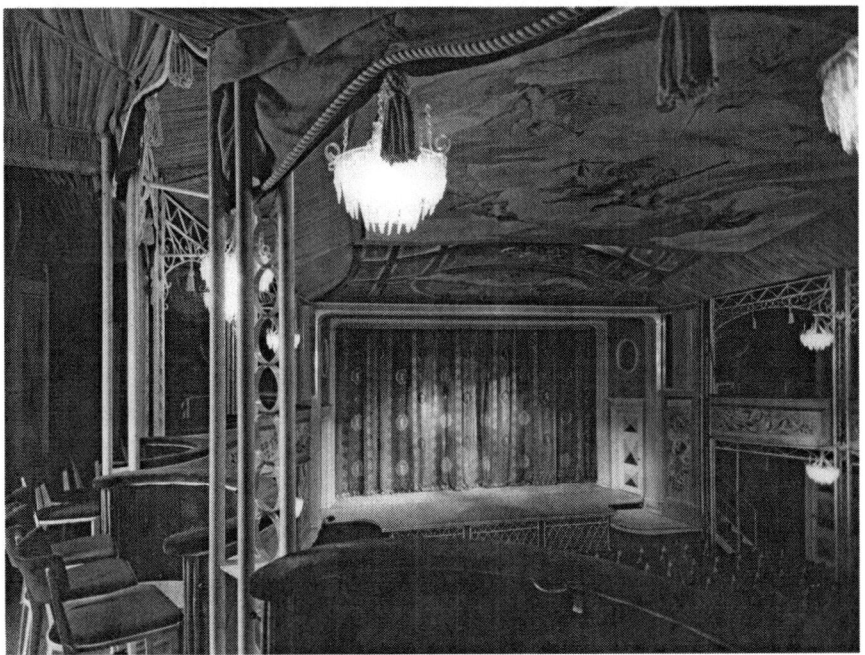

Interior of the Riverside Theatre, Battersea Pleasure Gardens, 1951, designed by the theatrical scenery designer Guy Sheppard and part-built by the Theatrical Scenery Construction firm of Brunskill and Loveday Limited. Photo: Courtesy of Brunskill and Loveday Limited, www.theatrical-scenery.info

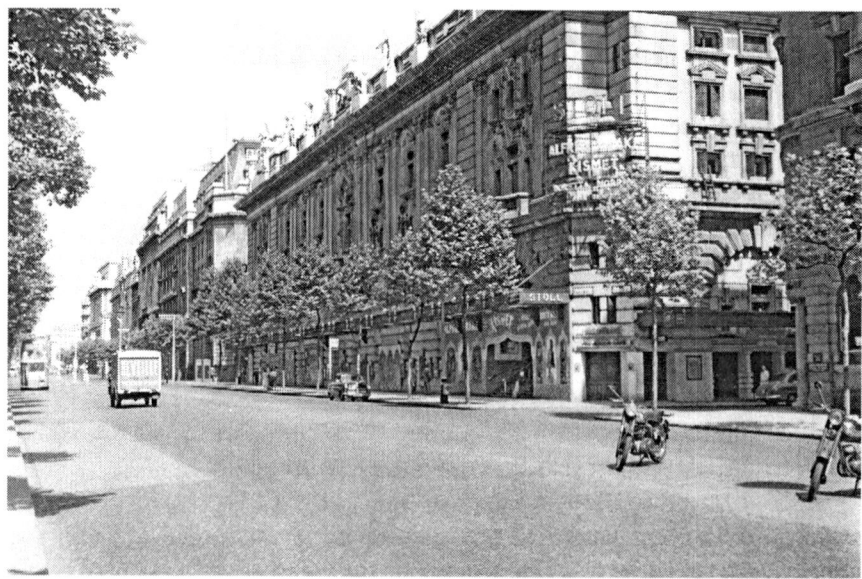

The Stoll Theatre from Kingsway, August Bank Holiday Monday, 1955. Photo: ©Courtesy of Allan Hailstone.

the 'terpsichorean delights' of Mister Sachs's Sylphides. This trio of dancers (Maria Sanina [Brigitte Kelly], Ann Wakefield and Lulu Dukes [daughter of Marie Rambert]), dressed à la Taglioni, are not showgirls, by any means. They have impeccable ballet backgrounds. They dance a 'Wedding Bouquet Ballet' and close the show with a can-can.[34] Here perhaps they dance of the pathos of the unmarried and unmarriageable, to that popular music hall theme of, 'Why am I always the bridesmaid, never the blushing bride?'[35]

Unlike the didactic national narrative of the South Bank Exhibition, and unlike the earnestness of the Arts Council's Festival of the Arts – opera, ballet, music, Shakespeare – the Pleasure Gardens offer a promenade of pick-and-mix popular taste, with rides, bandstands, acrobats, puppets, music and dancing. At the Pleasure Gardens, dance may be a pleasant trifle, but at least it is visible, and at the Amphitheatre a short ballet performance can be seen twice daily, six days a week for three months. There is also good, consistent work here for dancers. Dance in the Pleasure Gardens is knitted comfortably into the popular amusement of a population that needs to lap up diversion when it gets the opportunity.

The more upmarket Chelsea inhabitants of the north bank are also drawn to observe the shenanigans across the water. From Cheyne Walk and the Chelsea Embankment they can enjoy the floodlit view. Come across, the Pleasure Gardens make no class distinctions!

From the Stoll Theatre to the Royal Festival Hall

The Pleasure Gardens is not the Arts Council, which has a very different agenda. It is no surprise that the Arts Council's subsidised dance venues, the Royal Opera House Covent Garden and Sadler's Wells Theatre, are getting most attention for the London Festival of the Arts. But there is ballet in two other important venues. One is the Stoll Theatre, on Kingsway;[36] the other is the brand new Royal Festival Hall. The walk between the two theatres is significant, as much about movement in time from past to future as about southerly movement in space.

We begin on a wide, busy street of impressive buildings. Most impressive of all is the Stoll Theatre, a huge Edwardian edifice occupying a whole block on the eastern side of Kingsway, between Portugal Street and Sardinia Street. With an auditorium seating 2,600, it opened in 1911 as the London Opera House, a failed project of the first Oscar Hammerstein. In 1951 this is a prominent house that has presented all sorts of entertainments from opera to cinema, variety and ice shows. Viewing from the outside (and the opposite side of the street is best for this) there are large ornate windows at the upper level and a row of twelve statues by Thomas Rudge on the roof. At each end there are groups representing Melody and Harmony. The central figures of Inspiration and Composition are flanked by Comedy, Tragedy, Song and Dance.[37] The façade is said to be based on the Louvre in Paris and the interior is a riot of decoration, vaulted and domed, overflowing with baroque detailing of columns, arches, entablatures, roundels and swags, statuary and painted scenes of cherubs making music.[38] A reporter at Hammerstein's pre-opening open house gives some impressions of how it felt to enter the building.

> Entering by a broad flight of steps, we find ourselves in a large and convenient vestibule, on a level with 21 private boxes, two marble staircases leading down to the stalls, which are flanked on either side with more boxes, 16 in all. The stalls are placed on a very decided gradient, which allows everybody to have a remarkably good view of the stage; and the same principle has been observed throughout, so that in all parts of the house the view from the back seats will be uninterrupted.[39]

And the reporter at the opening performance reckoned that even for those who 'climbed other stairways into the well-planned balconies above... [t]here need to be no backaches or strained necks or cramped legs'.[40]

The Stoll's wide and deep stage makes it perfect for ballet, so it seems extraordinary that the first ballet company to perform here, in October 1950, was the new formation of a Markova-Dolin company now bearing the name

Festival Ballet. This is not to denote that it was formed solely for the Festival, but the company being in need of a name, and the word 'festival' being on everyone's lips, it seemed a wholly appropriate choice. The season was extended into January 1951 and the company is back here for two months from 7 May 1951 as part of the London Season of the Arts in honour of the Festival of Britain.

The lure of the partnership of Anton Dolin and Alicia Markova is historic, and strangely both nationalistic and cosmopolitan. Ballet enthusiasts attending a Markova-Dolin performance in 1951 are aware of the heritage embodied in these two stars. Both are British by birth[41] and now are the first British ballet stars with an international reputation from tours all over the Americas, western Europe, Australia and some parts of South-East Asia. In 1947 it is tendentious to bill them as 'The World's Greatest Ballet Stars'[42] but welcome of course as a counteractive to gloom over Britain's waning political power. Although British, they are impeccably qualified as inheritors of the Russian ballet tradition. Both students of the great Russian teacher in London, Serafina Astafieva, they were picked out in the 1920s by Serge Diaghilev to be part of his Ballets Russes company that made ballet a significant factor in London's theatrical life from 1911 until his death in 1929. Their 'Russified' names evoke that period when 'good ballet' meant Russian ballet. In the infant years of British ballet in the 1920s and 30s they lent their previous success to the development of British institutions of ballet but they were also intent on their own paths. In 1935 they formed their own company together, the Markova-Dolin Company.[43] Two years of touring spread their names around the country but by then it was time to go international in what was now the expanding scene of the marketable 'Ballet Russe' name. For the time being they signed with the two rival companies, Colonel de Basil's Ballets Russes and the Ballet Russe de Monte Carlo organised by René Blum. These companies inherited the mantle of Diaghilev in some of those old and loved productions, in the choreographers Fokine and Massine whose names will always be associated with Diaghilev, and in dancers of the older and new generation, many of whom literally represented the emigrated vestiges of Imperial Russia.[44] In 1951, the glow of celebrity that surrounds Markova and Dolin comes from exemplifying this tradition at source.

The outbreak of World War II isolated Markova and Dolin in America. It was not until 1948 that they were seen again in London as guests with the Sadler's Wells Ballet at Covent Garden. Still commercially bankable, they were able to fill huge London arenas at Earl's Court and Haringey in 1949.

By the time they get to the Stoll in 1951, Festival Ballet, based upon the partnership of Markova and Dolin, has reinforced its international reputation with a season at Monte Carlo and brought into its fold some of the

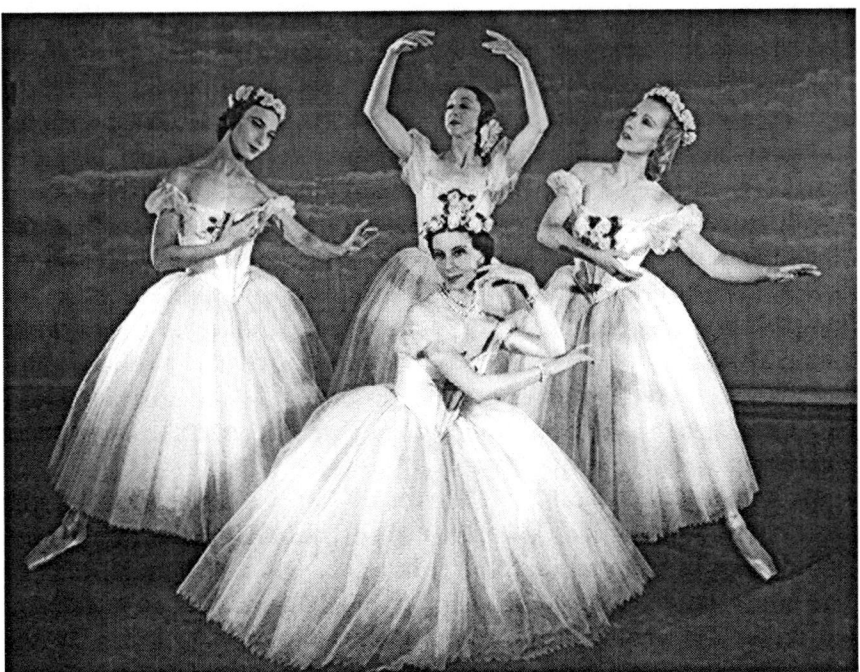

Pas de Quatre (chor. Dolin, 1941) in 1951, with (standing l. to r.) Nathalie Krassovska as Carlotta Grisi, Alexandra Danilova as Fanny Cerrito, Tatiana Riabouchinska as Lucile Grahn and (front) Alicia Markova as Marie Taglioni. Photo: © Baron/ Getty Images.

names from defunct or dying Ballets Russes companies. Nathalie Krassovska was with the Ballet Russe de Monte Carlo during the war years in America, personally having a special dedication to the ballets of Fokine. Nicholas Beriosoff brings his detailed knowledge of Petipa classics and his reputation for staging the Fokine Ballets Russes repertoire. A former 'baby ballerina', Tatiana Riabouchinska (one of the stars of de Basil's company aged just fifteen), and her choreographer husband, David Lichine, join for the season. Main guest artists are Alexandra Danilova, a star since her appearances with Diaghilev's company, and in the Ballet Russe successor companies and Mia Slavenska, who is also remembered from the Ballet Russe de Monte Carlo. This cluster of dancers epitomises the pleasures of the pre-war years of ballet-going for those who remember them: London summer seasons back in the 1930s; the rivalries between the companies, the ballerinas and their fans; the ballets of Balanchine, Fokine and Massine all with their direct heritage from Russia and Diaghilev.

The Festival Ballet repertoire this 1951 season includes Beriosoff's staging of *The Nutcracker* and the Fokine 'classics' from Diaghilev days of *Petrushka*, *Les Sylphides* and *Prince Igor* ('splendidly reproduced').[45] *Petrushka*, with its Stravinsky score and Benois designs is the very essence of the spirit of Diaghilev's Ballets Russes of long ago. Solo roles apart, we may wonder whether it is possible for the young British *corps de ballet* to understand and embody the crowd of the St Petersburg Shrovetide Fair as originally performed by Diaghilev's Russian dancers.[46] Fokine's atmospheric, *Spectre de la Rose*, difficult to recreate since it is always to be associated with the incomparable dancers Nijinsky and Karsavina who created it for Diaghilev in 1911, is newly admired in performances by Riabouchinska and the young British dancer, John Gilpin. Danilova as guest reprises her 1930s role of the Street Dancer in Massine's character ballet to the music of Johann Strauss, *Le Beau Danube*. Lionel Bradley is delighted to see her again. He thinks her 'long thin legs' are the most beautiful in ballet and she seems 'quite ageless' taking him back to when he first saw her perform the role. Markova's now legendary interpretation of *Giselle* is a major part of the programming.[47] New choreographies by resident choreographer David Lichine (*Impressions* and *Harlequinade*) are less well received.[48]

On 4 June four ballerinas – Markova, Danilova, Riabouchinska and Krassovska – perform Dolin's version of *Pas de Quatre*. This is the first London performance (it was premiered in America for Ballet Theatre in 1941).[49] This little ballet is many-faceted. Look at it in different lights or in different moods and its meaning dissolves and reforms into something else. On one level it is a sometimes crude attempt to imagine and recreate the occasion in 1845 when four of the most scintillating ballerinas of the romantic age – Marie Taglioni, Fanny Cerrito, Carlotta Grisi, and Lucile Grahn – were induced to perform together in London in a special choreography by Jules Perrot. This was one of the previous historical moments when London could be called a 'dance capital'. As these four ballerinas perform before us in 1951, is their embodiment of the roundness and softness of romantic era style unconvincing? Are attempts to dramatise the historic rivalry between them with exaggerated courtesies too much like caricature?[50] It is not to be taken as a literal historical document, at least not one about the nineteenth century. Much more, here in this programme, it suggests the return of the pre-war cosmopolitan ballet in the presence of these timeless ballerinas while they acknowledge the preeminent position of Markova, the English star.

The curtain rises on the recreation of Chalon's lithograph, the four ballerinas dressed in pale pink, garlanded with flowers. Markova as Taglioni stands centre, Krassovska as Grisi, Riabouchinska as Grahn and Danilova as Cerrito clustered around her. This is indeed like a garland of Russo-American flowers around the British *assoluta*. They dance a little together, sometimes making acknowledgement to Taglioni before three give the stage to Grahn for her solo. Now Riabouchinska shows her own qualities of lightness and speed. She ends with a long series of *entrechats*, up to thirty if possible, in which she changes front, raises her arms and fluffs her skirt, all as if to show there is no strain at all. The Grisi/Krassovska solo is next, witty, with stops and starts and *piqués*. Markova (Taglioni) and Riabouchinska (Grahn) now take to the stage, crossing and posing, finally making an arch through which Danilova as Cerrito emerges. In tradition, Cerrito is distinguished by not wearing the circlet of flowers that the other ballerinas are crowned with. A single, provocative rose is behind her ear, defining her as the contender for the ultimate crown of Taglioni. Her solo is in swooping waltz time, in which she indulges with deep body movements. She *jetés* off stage to great applause, returning to acknowledge her admirers before gesturing to her rival to begin. Now the Taglioni/Markova solo is a smooth and elegant contrast of a different kind of brilliance. She demonstrates her legendary balance in long, unsupported arabesques on *pointe*, seemingly to hover on air, finishing with fast footwork. It seems as if the legend of Markova merges with the legend of Taglioni.[51] Finally, all enter to dance together, rotating in a tight circle, kneeling, then rising to offer a few steps as individuals. They change places energetically across the circle with a hint of Spanish in their arms (you can hear the castanets in the music). In the last encircling of Markova, she seems veritably a reincarnation of Taglioni, kneeling serenely in front of them, forefinger delicately to her cheek. We all applaud like mad![52]

Here in the programming of Festival Ballet, *Pas de Quatre* speaks of a company that encompasses ballet's past as well as being graced by the presence of Markova. Even Danilova, who had ballerina status in Diaghilev's company (which Markova did not have), concedes the highest position to her. Danilova's time with Festival Ballet is marked by her generosity in passing on her heritage all the way from its Russian native roots. She teaches company class and coaches the young dancers in everything from mime to make-up. Lionel Bradley asks wistfully if he will ever see her dance again.[53] At her final performance, Markova herself presents the bouquet.

The season is marked out as a great success although some critical voices remark on the smallness of the repertoire and its predominant flavour of past times, rather than striving to develop new choreographic voices.[54]

*   *   *   *   *

Outside the Stoll, Kingsway is wide and straight. If it seems to us in 1951 to speak of solidity, tradition and a long history, this is the story it's meant to convey, but these neo-classical buildings lining the avenue are hardly fifty years old! The scheme that tore down the slums in its path drove Kingsway south, joining it to the Strand through the graceful curve of Aldwych. Its model was the Parisian boulevard but its meaning was imperial Britannia. Imperial London of 1905 was a different place to the London ruled by the Festival Star. Edward Elgar's wife wrote a poem, *The King's Way*, to celebrate its opening by King Edward VII in 1905, sung to a theme from Elgar's *Pomp and Circumstance March, No. 4.*

The noblest street in London town,
The Kingsway, the Kingsway!
The noblest street in London town,
The stir of life beats up and down;
In serried ranks the sabres shine,
And Art and Craft and Thought divine,
All crowd and fill the great highway,
The Kingsway, the Kingsway!

It's not great poetry, but its meaning is very clear – onwards, with monarchy and military to Empire! Built with an underground tramway coming back to the surface at Waterloo Bridge, Kingsway facilitated the journey to south of the Thames. In 1951 this is significant since it leads over Waterloo Bridge to the South Bank. As we walk, we may hear the rattle of trams underneath in the Kingsway tunnel. In twelve months these trams will have disappeared, and that will be progress![55] Turn right at the end of Kingsway and we are in Aldwych, almost immediately upon the palatial block with the Waldorf Hotel at its centre and a theatre at either end, the Aldwych and the Strand. Before turning left towards Waterloo Bridge, the huge columned portico of the Lyceum comes into view.[56] It's not a theatre; it hasn't been for some time, but a rather good ballroom. They've been trying something new here since May – professional male partners have been added to the female ones. Impeccable in evening dress, they have to sit in a pen waiting to be picked up for one shilling a dance, or thirty shillings for the whole evening. Perhaps it's embarrassment, or not a very 'British' idea but it has not been popular so far.[57] The Lyceum is also the scene of the annual Vic-Wells Ball, when dancers are allowed to abandon restraint and indulge in fantastical costuming for its own sake.[58]

Across Waterloo Bridge and amidst the activity of the South Bank Exhibition, International Ballet has the honour of being the first ballet company to perform in the Royal Festival Hall. The company, under its founder, director and *prima ballerina*, Mona Inglesby, is always admired for its persistence. Earlier in the year, International Ballet celebrated its tenth anniversary. Nobody denies that this is a considerable achievement for a company that started from scratch in the early war years and has since existed on constant touring, mainly outside London, without public subsidy. As well as London and provincial theatres, it has played some of the 'super cinema' stages like the huge Gaumont State at Kilburn, brought the ballet classics to large audiences to whom they were a new experience and instituted educational programmes. They have even performed at a Butlin's holiday camp. All of this is much admired even though the repertoire is short and dominated by the classics.[59] It is Inglesby's personal crusade to have these staged with the greatest authenticity according to the Stepanov system notations in the possession of her émigré Russian ballet master, Nicolai Sergeyev, whose death in June this year is a blow to her.[60] So *Swan Lake, Giselle, Coppélia,* and *The Sleeping Princess* are central to her repertoire with a few new choreographies, her own production of the *Everyman* morality play, for instance.[61] There is also acknowledgement of the early twentieth century. Last year Massine staged for them his *demi-caractère* ballets from the Ballet Russe de Monte Carlo, *Gaîeté Parisienne* and *Capriccio Espagñol.* They have some Fokine ballets from the Diaghilev era, *Les Sylphides* and *Carnaval.*

It is perhaps to be expected that we all focus on the venue. Just to step inside is to wonder at its openness and airiness. This is a world away from the ornately effusive decoration at the Stoll or Covent Garden. The foyers and stairways are wide, with walls of glass and there are terraces for taking the air during intervals. Light and air is a feature of the auditorium with its pale wood panelling and boxes that seem to float gently out of the walls. Everyone has a perfect view from the raked seating, all above stage level. It isn't loved by everybody of course: Peter Williams calls it 'a tricked up aeroplane-hangar'.[62]

It is certainly a disaster for ballet, built as a concert hall without proscenium, and probably never envisaged as a theatre. For a company director who values above all the theatrical impact of spectacle with all its possibilities of lighting and stage setting[63] this venue seems a strange choice. Perhaps the issue is more about Inglesby's other agenda of presenting ballet to new audiences – ballet to the masses. Special tickets are available that include a ballet matinée with entry to the South Bank Exhibition at 10.30 am. An evening ticket for 8 pm allows entrance to the Festival grounds at 7.15 and to remain until the end of proceedings at 11 pm.

International Ballet's advertising explains that the presentation will be: '[a] system of "light-décor" specially designed to harmonize with the atmosphere and mood of the different ballets and the architectural character of the Hall.'[64] In practice, the permanent setting resembles a terraced garden: grass on the steps, hedges, and bits of masonry, used with minor adaptations for all the ballets. The stage built over the orchestra area sounds hollow, and makes footfall in *pointe* shoes very loud. Entrances and exits have to be made through arches at either side and down flights of steps in full audience view, even causing some nasty slips on the fake grass. It's light and air taken to excess, almost like an open-air performance.

> Those star entrances and exits so beloved of ballerinas and balletomanes are out of the question at the Festival Hall. There is no thrilling leap into the wings after a variation. Instead, the artist has to climb the grassy steps, and often the applause has died away before the dancer has managed to get out of sight.... The ballerina is always seen to better

advantage behind a magic row of glowing footlights and framed by elegant pillars and rich crimson curtains.[65]

The premiere of the season, a ballet by Harcourt Algeranoff, *For Love or Money*, has a story that is far too complicated and ends up being quite a muddle.[66] So despite the courage in getting ballet right into the centre of the most iconic British event since the end of the war, this is not a critical success for International Ballet. On the other hand the houses are full and appreciative. There might be something worthwhile in taking ballet to the South Bank after all!

July 1951
26th : Korean ceasefire talks begin.

August
21st : Death of Constant Lambert, musical director of Sadler's Wells Ballet.
25th : A civil defence exercise in Southampton simulates a raid on the city. 1,400 troops and 200 vehicles take part.
31st : First long-playing record launched in Germany.

To Seven Dials via Drury Lane and Leicester Square

In terms of location, this walk begins at Waterloo Bridge and moves in a generally north westerly direction. In terms of dance it moves through musical theatre, film, variety and 'foreign' dance companies.

Up past the Lyceum is the famous Theatre Royal Drury Lane. Diaghilev's Ballets Russes performed here in 1913 and 1914, and in 1938 the Ballet Russe de Monte Carlo was here, while its rival, the Original Ballet Russe, performed at Covent Garden and fans nipped between the theatres during intervals to catch their favourites. Since 1947 it has been the home of two of the American musicals with integrated plot enhancing ballets, first *Oklahoma!* and now *Carousel* is coming to the end of its long run. Both of these have Agnes de Mille's choreography. Some remember her as a dancer with Ballet Rambert and Antony Tudor's Dance Theatre in London in the 1930s, but she was just a visitor then and now we can see the real American identity in her style. Her Americana ballet *Rodeo* and the psychological, 'state of mind' piece, *Fall River Legend* (about the Lizzie Borden axe murders in Massachusetts, 1892) were danced here in 1950 by the American Ballet Theatre. She seems to have absorbed an eclectic mix of training, including the American modern dance with its concern for the inner motivation of a character. Dance in musical theatre has been changed by productions such as *Oklahoma!* and *Carousel*. Choreography now can advance the plot rather than being a decorative pause. British choreographers try to emulate her, but with little success so far. Is ballet training now proved insufficient for the new kind of stage musical? Where will the new kind of modern dance come from? [67]

In *Carousel* the dance scenes are all about feelings. At the end of 'June is bustin' out all over' there is breathy elation, being young and smelling love in the air. In the 'Hornpipe', you can feel the sexual tension between the young women and the sailors who taunt the girls with 'Release your davits and jump'. The 'Beach Ballet' introduces the daughter of Julie and the deceased Billy for the first time, as a lonely adolescent who plays with the 'Badly Brought up Boys' because the Snow family snubs her. She is attracted and rejected by some passing carnival people and 'A Young Man like Billy'. The ballet danced barefoot by Louise, fully fleshes out the rebellious, passionate and obstinate character, so that the only line, 'I hate you, all of you', seems superfluous. Rambert's former ballerina, Sally Gilmour took over the role of Louise from Bambi Linn with great success in 1950 .[68] This proves that British dancers are capable of this transition, whatever Hanya Holm may say (see page 7).

To reach Leicester Square we can cut through Covent Garden Market, avoiding the stray residues of vegetables in the gutters (for this is still a wholesale fruit, vegetable and flower market). Close to the Coliseum (where another American musical, *Kiss Me Kate* is playing) we cross St Martin's Lane and then Charing Cross Road. Leicester Square is a centre for film with two major cinemas, the Odeon and the Empire used for royal film command performances. Having just considered the demand for modern dance technique in musical theatre, it becomes quite interesting that there are two films doing the rounds this summer of 1951 in which ballet, proper ballet with well-formed technique, has a major part. These films are opposites on a number of levels: one British, one American; one made in Shepperton, Surrey, one from Hollywood, California.

Premiered in April at the Carlton on the Haymarket, *The Tales of Hoffmann*, is a Powell and Pressburger film aiming to follow up on the huge success of *The Red Shoes* (1948) with some of the same team. Again the Sadler's Wells Ballet principal Moira Shearer is the ballerina. Robert Helpmann and Léonide Massine are the principal male actor/dancers and Frederick Ashton is choreographer and performer. With Shearer, Helpmann and Ashton (resident choreographer of Sadler's Wells Ballet) and supporting dancers there is a strong British dance contingent and many of our favourite dancers are here. That is something to be proud of in a feature film.

The Red Shoes was a story *about* ballet, and about the possessive demands placed on the ballerina by the company director, who seems to be based on Diaghilev. There is a ballet scene at the heart of the film, intended to be understood both as a real ballet performance in a theatre and a metaphorical exploration of the state of mind of Shearer's character, torn between her career and personal happiness. *The Tales of Hoffmann* is quite different, a filmed opera by Offenbach (1881) with dancing interpolated in a somewhat

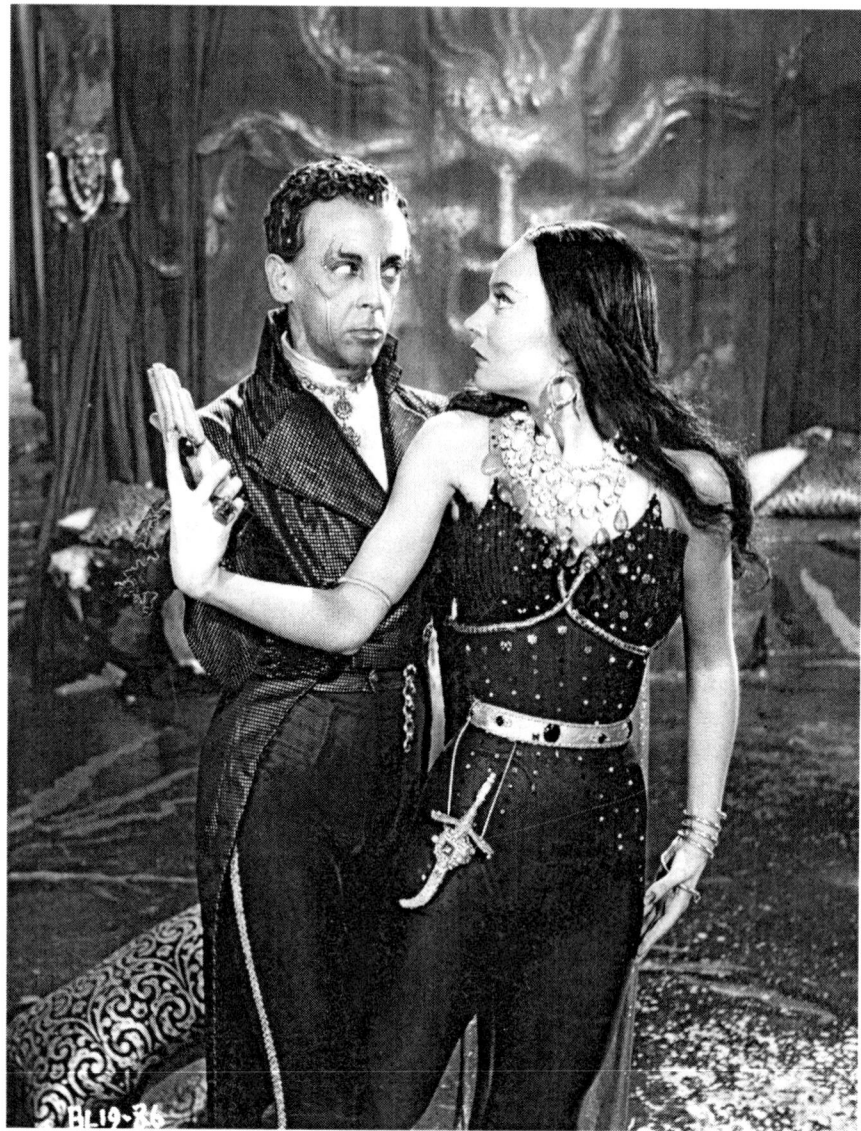

Robert Helpmann as Dr Dapertutto with Ludmilla Tcherina as Giulietta in *Tales of Hoffmann* (Powell and Pressburger, 1951). © Hulton Archive/Getty Images.

haphazard way. It definitely interests today's ballet audiences as these tales are the root of the 1870 ballet *Coppélia*. The first of the *Tales*, is about Olympia who is an automaton as is the doll in *Coppélia* but the Coppelius in *Hoffmann* is a maker of magic spectacles and eyes, rather than the harmless doll-maker of the ballet.

Dancers mime their roles taken by opera singers on the sound track which looks unconvincing. While the setting is supposed to be in the nineteenth century, historical and locational realities are not consistent. For example Shearer appears in 'The Enchanted Dragonfly Ballet' in the Prologue, clad in all-over tights, while in the Epilogue Ballet she is dressed in a 'sylphide' length tutu. Most actors have costumes with some approximation to the nineteenth century. Perhaps the contradictions don't matter since this is essentially a fantasy. The three stories have malign fate and magic at their core and, as soon as Hoffmann embarks upon the tales, reality is abandoned anyway.

Each of the three tales takes place in a different fictional space and although it's clear that this is a sound-stage, the action feels very theatrical apart from a few uses of split screen and interesting dissolves. It's no surprise that this is the vision of a theatrical designer Hein Heckroth. In 'Olympia' acres of silks and gauzes are used to deepen and divide the space for separate scenes. Lighting and backgrounds are strongly coloured with purple, gold, orange and yellow, decorated by unsettling images – eyes, masks. An unrolled carpet makes a fictive staircase. There is even a follow-spot. In 'Giulietta' the gondola floats on lighting effects like painted water. Coloured candle drippings of green, blue and red are turned into gems. It's visually lush, although some find it garish and the mix altogether too indigestible, overloaded with decoration.[69]

In each act Helpmann is the variously named magician who conspires to bring down Hoffmann and his is undoubtedly the most successful acting. His mastery of the ironic eyebrow lift is unsurpassed. Every deceitful thought shows in his face. His Coppelius is crazy and uncontrolled. His Lindorf and Dapertutto are studied malevolence. Massine seems less comfortable in his roles: his Spalanzani like a reprise of the Peruvian in *Gaîeté Parisienne*. Of the choreography, the dance Ashton created for Shearer as the mechanical doll, Olympia, is most effective, full of variety and interesting complexities of sequences; however you have to suspend belief that she can pirouette, *jeté* and *fouetté* so consummately while singing too!

'Hoffmann' is a contribution to the Festival of Britain and the literal demonstration of that is when the final frames show a hand appearing to stamp on the back of the music score, 'Made in England'. Monica sees the film on 17 May.

Now in August in Leicester Square we can see that other film, *An American in Paris* with Gene Kelly. The Square has been a centre of theatreland since the mid-nineteenth century, with a long rivalry between the biggest theatres, the Empire and the Alhambra (new replaced by the Odeon Cinema). Their music hall ballet companies from the 1860s until shortly before World War I were central to what ballet in London was in those days: if highly-developed technique was limited to foreign ballerinas, the spectacle was everything. The Empire is the second theatre of that name on this plot. Strangely enough, there is once more a company here called the Empire Ballet. The film will be part of a hybrid presentation called cine-variety. A fifty minute stage show precedes the film and it all happens four times daily! It says 'Showplace of the Nation' on its programmes and this is a splendid revival of the kind of show incorporating film that used to be common, even until quite recently.

This week the stage show is topical. It starts as usual with the Empire Grand Organ. Then there is the second edition of the variety show called *Festival* that plays off the current Festival of Britain. It starts with a dancing and singing scene with the Empire Singers and the Empire Ballet called 'Come to Britain', not exactly the official Festival song of 'All the World is Coming to London', but reflecting it in gusto. A few weeks ago they promised an aeroplane on stage, bringing visitors to the South Bank, but instead we have 'Airborne Precision' from the Empire Girls, a line of 24 high kickers, supposedly set on the South Bank. Then the Empire Orchestra and the Empire Chorus in a stage set that looks like the Concert Pavilion from Battersea Pleasure Gardens give a medley from the British hit parade. They have an amazing device, a kind of trolley-lift that moves the orchestra from the pit to the stage without them ever stopping playing or changing seats! The Three Wilkes do their trapeze act, 'Thrills and Spills', just like the acts at the Lakeside in the Pleasure Gardens. The Empire Ballet performs a 'Souvenir of 1897', choreographed by Alan Carter, a little vignette of a family visiting the Crystal Palace during Queen Victoria's Diamond Jubilee Celebrations. Balancing acts and a comedian make up the section called 'Festival Fun'. The finale with the whole cast is called 'Britannia on Holiday'.[70] This stage show may be one of the best yet at the Empire and Carter's ballet is highly successful and appropriate for dancers and audience.[71]

An American in Paris makes some attempt to claim contemporaneity. The hero, Jerry Mulligan (Gene Kelly) is a former G.I. trying to make his way as a painter in postwar Paris, and his love interest, Lise (Leslie Caron) finds it difficult to reject her other suitor, who sheltered her during the war while her parents were in the Resistance. Caron is remembered in London as a very young dancer with Les Ballets des Champs Elysées at its second London season in 1949 and particularly in her role of the Sphinx in David Lichine's Oedipus ballet, *La Rencontre*.[72]

In contrast to *Hoffmann's* fantasy staging, there seems to be a superficial reality in Kelly's Paris streets. There is a family café, a cheap garret, a Parisian *perfumier*, the bank of the Seine, all looking exactly as you would expect them in real life, so it is a shock to learn they were all created on set in Hollywood. But when the film is called on to make thoughts, dreams and fears visual, it makes full use of cinematic techniques. So the description of Lise in her varying moods gives Caron a series of ballet solos using split screen, Jerry's pianist friend imagines performing at a concert, conducting

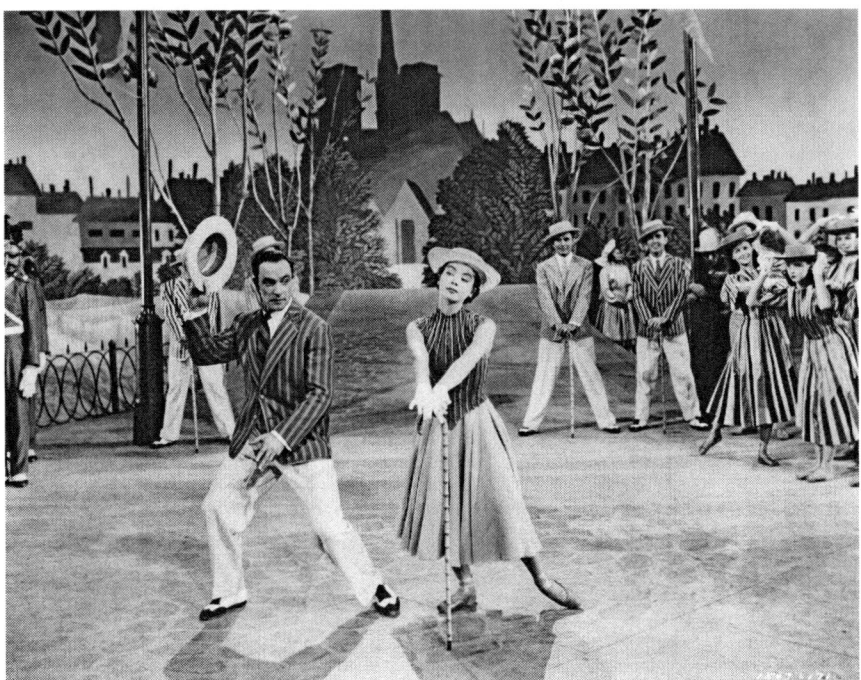

Gene Kelly and Leslie Caron in *An American in Paris* (dir. Minnelli, 1951). Photo: © John Springer Collection/CORBIS

and playing all the instruments too. Then the film reaches its conclusion in a long ballet scene set to a new arrangement (and sometimes dis-arrangement) of Gershwin's *An American in Paris*.[73] It supposedly happens in Jerry's head while he believes he has just lost Lise for good. This is a literal playing out of the title, since we have an American, Kelly (but others too, if we count Gershwin and other American characters who appear), situated in scenes that evoke and directly quote the Paris of painters Dufy, Renoir, Utrillo, Henri Rousseau and Toulouse Lautrec.[74] Unlike the gaudy colours of *Tales of Hoffmann*, Kelly's ballet plays with the subtle colour contrasts of the painters, sometimes fading to monochrome.

Throughout the ballet Jerry is always finding and losing Lise. Their first encounter is in the Place de la Concorde as expressed by Dufy. Next, in a flower market inspired by Renoir, they meet and he supports her in a tender *pas de deux*, but finds himself alone again in a Paris street scene by Utrillo. Now he is joined by four fellow Americans in uniform. Preparing to take the city by storm, they drag him into the group: it's almost going to be a classic American buddy movie like *On the Town*. They get hold of some dandified 'civvy' clothes, blazers, canes and straw hats. Now, more than ever they are 'in Paris', dressed as *boulevardiers* (Maurice Chevalier comes to mind). We follow some French guardsmen into a new part of town, with trees and

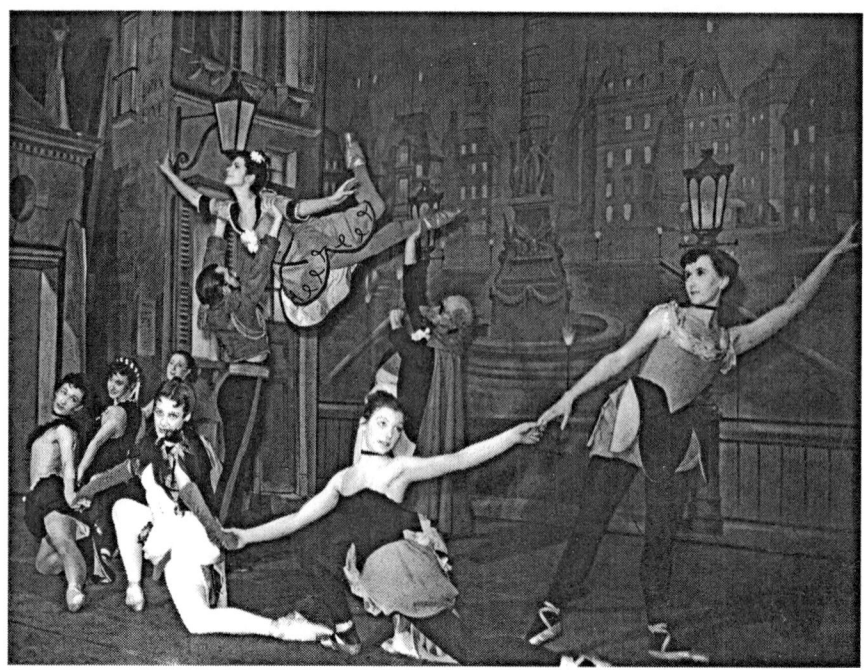

Absinthe Frappé (chor. Frank Staff) performed by the Empire Ballet in the stage show *Cheers*, accompanying the film *Adam's Rib* (dir. Cukor) at the Empire Cinema, Leicester Square, February 1950. (Staff preceded Alan Carter as ballet master at the Empire). Photographer not credited.

zoo animals treated in the *naïf* style of Rousseau. Lise is here amongst an ensemble of girls, 'chic', excitable, flirtatious. They are all on *pointe*, with delicately *piqué* -ing steps and they finish up with a whole flurry of *fouettés*. The Americans arrive on the scene, straw hats aloft, showing off their tap dancing, '*la danse Americaine*'. The scene ends with all the characters, including guardsmen and *mesdemoiselles,*the latter on *pointe*, joining in their 'yankee doodle strut' (a staccato straight-legged walk with body leaning forward).[75] So this gives America a temporary victory. The ballet ends as it began, all dancing in Dufy's representation of La Place de la Concorde with its central fountain before everyone except Jerry suddenly disappears from the scene.

This show raises questions, particularly with the memory of *Tales of Hoffman* earlier in the year. *American in Paris* seems so sophisticated in comparison and not only in its cinematic techniques.[76] The choreography and music shift between different styles, but always inflected with jazz rhythms to some degree and the ballet sequences seem to be configured for a more eclectic style, each dance technique (tap, ballet, can-can, jazz dance) blended together and used to its own best effect. There is an energy and pace throughout that contrasts with how slowly *Hoffmann* moves along. It is doubtful whether *Hoffmann*, could make new converts for either opera or ballet, whereas *An American in Paris* is very persuasive about the power of dance to communicate wordlessly. Seen as part of a cine-variety programme, with Part I a conventional variety show set in London and Part II a new form of musical film set in Paris, it is the latter that seems most appealingly contemporary.

But wait: let's examine this in another light! Cine-variety is not just an outmoded genre known only here in Britain. Somehow this show at the Empire is much more complicated. This has been instigated by American cinema giant Metro Goldwyn Mayer to replicate in its principal cinema in London the shows put on in their Radio City Music Hall in New York. 'Showcase of the Nation' is also the Radio City's banner. Producer Nat Karson and chorus line choreographer, Edward Noll, have been brought in from New York. At Radio City the scale is grander but there, just as here, there is a ballet company alongside its Rockettes chorus line.[77] Certainly, quite apart from its thematic material, the Empire Ballet has an all-British flavour, choreographed by Alan Carter who, after a period in Sadler's Wells Theatre Ballet, was director of the St James's Ballet, and ballet-master/performer in *The Red Shoes* and *Tales of Hoffman*. Other names in the cast are known from established British ballet companies, no doubt bringing with them the styles they have previously trained and performed in.[78] So it seems that something of an amalgamation is going on at the Empire, between the production techniques of New York and the performance styles of the British dancers.[79]

*   *   *   *   *

The route to Seven Dials goes up the Charing Cross Road, past no.75 where Cyril Beaumont still has his famous bookshop and the little back room where dancers often go to study the history of their roles. Seven Dials was laid out in the 1690s as seven streets around a central gathering place with a column. It seems that the area has always been fighting for its reputation. Its name was synonymous with one of the Rookeries of nineteenth century London, but it appears that the worst slums were further north than the meeting point of the roads and they were swept away by the building of New Oxford Street. The original pillar was dismantled in 1773 and re-erected in Weybridge in 1820 as a monument to the Duchess of York, a local benefactor. In the twentieth century Seven Dials suffers from having a less recognisable ambiance than its neighbours. Seemingly it cannot live up to the seaminess of Soho to the west, to the cabbages and culture of Covent Garden Market to the east, or to the thriving theatreland of Shaftesbury Avenue to its north. This may have an effect on the fortunes of the Cambridge Theatre, built in 1930 at the apex of the triangle between Earlham Street and Mercer Street.

But there is something magical about this point of confluence at the centre of a star. If we want to look for urban ley-lines, perhaps this would be the place.[80]

The original interior decoration of the theatre was 'dusky pink contrasted with pale blue and silver'.[81] In 1951 we are seeing the recent redecoration in 'a ghastly salmon-red paint-out and a jumble of unsuitable light fittings'.[82] But perhaps this matters little now when pre-war taste is looking weary. In 1951 the Cambridge Theatre is about to become the theatrical hub of impresario Peter Daubeny's enterprise to bring overseas productions to London, which will entail the promotion of dance companies from abroad for a number of years. Daubeny is capitalising on London's current fascination for Spanish dancing. There have already been visits by Carmen Amaya's troupe (who set up a gypsy family headquarters in a café near Shaftesbury Avenue)[83], and Teresa and Luisillo, a Mexican couple, performing at the Stoll[84] and also in the suburbs, where Monica sees them at the Streatham Hill Theatre.

The first Daubeny production is to be Rosario and Antonio from June to July 1951, never before seen on a London stage but with a mammoth reputation, one performance on BBC television[85] and a season at the Edinburgh Festival. When Daubeny succeeds in bringing them to the Cambridge Theatre, Richard Buckle has already praised Antonio as one of the two or three best male dancers in the world[86] and this soon gets translated into 'the greatest dancer of our time'.[87] The day before his opening, Antonio is taken to see Festival Ballet at the Stoll Theatre and is photographed with Anton Dolin on the stage. Rosario and Antonio, 'The Kids from Seville', are hugely successful in London, with a repertoire including flamenco and other regional Spanish dances and some from Latin America. Rosario sings in a husky, soulful voice. Antonio dances some of his free choreography to Spanish composers (Turina, Granados, Soler). Most of all he is celebrated for his *Zapateado* to the music of Sarasate. This is the absolute pinnacle of his art, in stunningly differentiated flamenco footwork, seeming to concern a heroic struggle against great odds. As Buckle colourfully explains, he is like 'a gallant and beautiful messenger on horseback...dangerous descents, steady climbs and breathtaking leaps across chasms, arriving at last in a glow of physical well-being, to fling down a royal reprieve with a flourish... at some grim gaoler's feet'.[88] Monica sees him on 21 June and pronounces his *Zapateado* 'Miraculous'. With exiled Spaniards shouting their greetings and approval from the balcony, before, mid and after dances, this is almost like being in Spain![89] Lionel Bradley finds the whole evening 'a crescendo of delight'. Antonio does not have the same 'animal vitality and attractiveness' as Luisillo but he has 'real nobility of carriage, a sly wit and sense of humour'. Of his *Zapateado*, it reaches 'a new standard' in dynamic range, light and shade.[90] The spell cast by the performance spreads the atmosphere of *feria* out into the London night, says Elsa Brunelleschi.

Can you not see the balloons and orange blossom hanging from the balconies? Those salty morsels at the corner of Earlham street – yes – they are shrimps from the Guadalquivir and the ruddy cheeks behind the kiosk, of course, they really belong to an olive-skinned Gipsy, proffering sticky sweets and hot fried doughnuts. Let us walk in the cinnamon-scented air to the *Taberna* down the street, we shall celebrate with the *cañas* of Manzanilla. But we are in London, you say – in Seven Dials, not Seville, although we have just been watching Rosario and Antonio dancing *Sevillanas*.[91]

Daubeny follows on with further dance companies in the same theatre: Ballets des Champs Elysées in August,[92] Pilar Lopez (sister of La Argentinita) and Company in September[93], Le Grand Ballet du Marquis de Cuevas in October,[94] Mrinalini Sarabhai from October into November,[95] followed by a second season of Rosario and Antonio from November into December.[96] This flurry of activity feeds London's appetite, not only for ballet but also for dance from other cultures, particularly Indian and Spanish. Apart from Daubeny's projects, there are other imports during 1951: Ram Gopal in January and a Swedish Ballet Company in February, African-American Pearl Primus at the Princes Theatre in October, Uday Shankar in December and the final attempt to resuscitate the Original Ballet Russe after the death of Colonel de Basil at the Royal Festival Hall in December. Most significantly, rival Spanish dancers José Greco and Company appear at Sadler's Wells in June and July[97] leading to some partisanship amongst commentators. Who is better, Greco or Antonio? Greco is Italian, so is his dancing inauthentic? Battle lines are drawn in the press.[98]

To the river!

Wherever we are, at nights out in the summer of 1951 – Covent Garden, Drury Lane, the Stoll, the Cambridge, the Empire – we are all drawn in the end to look at the South Bank before we go home. We can just linger and listen. The bands play. The people dance out in the open! And watch: there are fireworks, and gas jets gush out through the fountains at the end of the Fairway. A fanciful bit of reportage says:

> Flowers of Fire that Bloom When the Moon Rises: Reality is dissolved in fancy, common-sense routed in poetical confusion. Water spouts into fronds of flame. Light flows in shimmering rivers. Steel and concrete take on the delicacy of gold and silver filigree, the city's skyline arcs into a thousand fantastic rainbows.'[99]

The Skylon, lit from inside and the Dome of Discovery, lit from underneath, seem to hover just above the ground, vertical and horizontal cyphers of newness and modernity when London's dark years are so recent.

On closing night, 29 September, there is dancing in three areas of the Exhibition until a quarter to midnight. Long into the night there is community singing. On Sunday morning, 30 September the flag is ceremoniously lowered. Within a month, the Labour government that gave birth to the Festival will have been defeated in a General Election and the scrapping will begin.

September 1951
23rd : King George VI has an operation for lung cancer.
29th: Closure of the South Bank Exhibition. Pleasure Gardens remain open.

October
3rd : British workers evacuated from the oil refinery at Abadan, Iran, shutting facility. Western boycotts cause Iranian crisis.
5th : Sadler's Wells Theatre Ballet opens its first north American tour in Quebec.
6th : Assassination of the British High Commissioner in Malaya by communist guerrillas at height of Malay Emergency.
13th : A new transmitter at Holm Moss, Yorkshire, brings television to the north of England.
25th : General Election won by Conservative Party. Winston Churchill becomes Prime Minister.

At the year's end it is possible to write, 'Indeed, if Festival Year is remembered at all in the annals of the theatre, it will surely be because of the flood of ballet and dance companies and recitals we have seen.'[100] With all this, 1951 is perhaps the high point of the impression that London is 'the dancing capital of the world'.[101] Dance companies from across the globe crave the approbation of London audiences.[102] Surely the future is bright!

Notes

1 'The Great Art of London', from *Things Near and Far* (1923) as reproduced in *The Collected Arthur Machen*, Christopher Palmer, ed. (1988), pp. 322-324.

2 'Introduction: Later Housing and its Contexts' (2008), in *The Survey of London, vol. 47, Northern Clerkenwell and Pentonville*, available from 'Introduction', Survey of London: volume 47: Northern Clerkenwell and Pentonville (2008), pp. 1-21. URL: http://www.british-history.ac.uk/source.aspx?pubid=1287.

3 'Merrie Islington', *The Evening News*, 11 July 1914, as reprinted in *The Collected Arthur Machen*, p.345.

4 I take this name and date from *The Survey of London*, vol. 47, Ch. V (2008) which discusses common mistakes over Sadler's name in relation to the evidence.

5 The frieze is now inside the entrance to the Lilian Baylis Theatre at Sadler's Wells.

6 See: 'Bevin Court, Holford House and Amwell House', in *Survey of London*, vol. 47, Ch. IX, Percy Circus Area.

7 Lionel Bradley, Ballet Bulletins, 21 February 1951. Theatre Collection, Victoria and Albert Museum.

8 Collingwood was sparing in comments written on her programmes, generally offering only a word of appreciation.
9 Mary Clarke, *Ballet Today*, May 1951, p.12.
10 The Sitter Out, *The Dancing Times*, May 1951, p.452.
11 Director-General of the Festival of Britain, Gerald Barry, text of press conference, 14 October 1948.
12 Music arranged by Charles Mackerass. The story is freely based upon the verses of *The Bumboat Woman's Story* by W.S. Gilbert and bears some resemblance to the plot of Gilbert and Sullivan's *H.M.S. Pinafore.*
13 His most famous invention is Maudie Littlehampton in a cartoon in the *Daily Express*. She is an aristocratic hangover from pre-war, trying to make sense of new times.
14 This is how the female *corps de ballet* is named in the cast list.
15 Analysis of *Pineapple Poll* is based upon two BBC transmissions: Production by Margaret Dale (1959) with the Royal Ballet (Merle Park and David Blair); Production by Bob Lockyer (1979) with the Sadler's Wells Royal Ballet (Marion Tait and Desmond Kelly).
16 Designed by Abram Games.
17 'The Sitter Out', *The Dancing Times*, May 1951, pp. 452-453.
18 L.J 'Call Pineapple Poll', undated press cutting in Monica Collingwood Collection, Tower Bridge Scrapbook No. 1. 'Lord Festival' became a popular nickname for the Labour politician Herbert Morrison whose correct title was Lord President of the Council, since he presided at the monarch's Privy Council. Morrison had Cabinet responsibility for the Festival of Britain.
19 Bradley, Ballet Bulletins, 11 April 1951. There are signs that he was already experiencing ill-health and he died peacefully on New Year's Eve 1953.
20 *The Festival of Britain 1951: the Official Book of the Festival of Britain.*
21 See: R.D. Russell and Robert Gooden (1976) 'The Lion and Unicorn Pavilion', in Mary Banham and Bevis Hillier eds. *A Tonic to the Nation: The Festival of Britain 1951*, pp.96-101.
22 A.P. Herbert, 'Welcome the World!' from *Festival Pleasure Gardens: Official Guide*, pp.11-12.
23 John Piper thought of his design as a folly. Banham and Hillier eds.(1976) *A Tonic to the Nation: The Festival of Britain 1951*, p.124.
24 In the Museum of London's collection of memories of the Festival, a number of participants, children at the time, recall the power of the Grotto and its perfumes.
25 John Dilworth, 'Festival Dance Pavilion', *The Dancing Times*, July 1951, p.619.
26 For example: for Ballet Rambert, *Lady into Fox* (1939), *The Sailor's Return* (1947); for London Ballet, later in Ballet Rambert repertory, *La Fête étrange* (1940); for Sadler's Wells Theatre Ballet, *Assembly Ball* (1946).
27 I include: Joy Carter, John Hall, Sonya Hana, Elizabeth Schooling, Robin Winbow, Jack Carter, Peter Darrell.
28 'The Sitter Out', *The Dancing Times*, July 1951, pp.579 – 580. See also Peter Williams, 'Orlando's Silver Wedding', *Dance and Dancers*, August 1951, p.15; 'Festival Gardens', *The Times*, 20 July 1951, p.8; 'Battersea Park', *The Stage*, 31 May, 1951, p.10.
29 Ballet Bulletins, 22 June 1951. He also saw it on 15 June after the performance of Balinese dance at the Riverside Theatre.
30 'Battersea Gardens: The Lambeth Walkers', *The Stage*, 31 May 1951, p.4.
31 Don Burland, 'The Riverside Theatre', *Illustrated London News*, 2 June 1951, pp.25, 32. I have not been able to trace any use of the Riverside Theatre after 1952. It appears that it was sent for scrap!

32 Ballet Bulletins, 15 June, 1951. Liong Sie wrote about Indonesian dance, 'Back to Bali', *Dance and Dancers*, June 1951, pp.9, 11, with illustrations of their two dances, *Baris Kembar* and *Tjalonarang*. The Sie siblings studied modern dance and Balinese dance in their native Java and later studied ballet with Borovansky in Australia and Idzikowsky in London. They were said to perform 'balletesque' versions of Balinese dances (Matthew Isaac Cohen, 2010, *Performing Otherness: Java and Bali on International Stages*, p.213). Edo Sie eventually became a flamenco dancer and was still teaching in Chicago in 2006 (Jeffrey Felshman, 'Long Lives: The Devil made him do it', *Chicago Reader*, 13 January 2006, pp. 12-13, available from : http://www.chicagoreader.com/pdf/060113/060113_wearing.pdf accessed 29 October 2012.

33 The format transferred to the BBC, televised from the City Varieties, Leeds, with Sachs as Chairman, broadcast from 1953-1983.

34 'Battersea Park', *The Stage*, 31 May, 1951, p.10. I have not been able to discover any further evidence about the Wedding Bouquet Ballet. Brigitte Kelley's autobiographical essays mention working for the Players Theatre and at Riverside Theatre, but she does not describe this show. See: (1999) 'Dancing for Joy: A Memoir Part Three', *Dance Chronicle*, vol.22, no.3, pp.408-410. Her memory is that the bad weather that summer made for very poor audiences.

35 Music hall artiste Lily Morris sings it on www.britishpathe.com *The Singing Cinema*.

36 This theatre was demolished in 1958. The site is now occupied by an office block with the Peacock Theatre in its basement.

37 'The New London Opera House', *The Times*, 1 August 1911, p. 10.

38 For the background to the purchase by Oscar Hammerstein, see: Vincent Sheean (1956) *Oscar Hammerstein I: The Life and Exploits of an Impresario*.

39 'The London Opera House: Mr. Hammerstein's New Building', *The Times*, 28 October 1911, p.8.

40 'The London Opera House: Opening Performance', *The Times*, 14 November 1911, p.11.

41 Their real names were Lilian Alicia Marks and Patrick Healy-Kay. Dolin was Irish by heritage but born in England.

42 As billed for their tours managed by Julian Braunsweg.

43 They were managed by Vivian Van Damm and financed by the Mrs Laura Henderson, owner of the Windmill Theatre. They rehearsed at the Windmill but did not perform there as has erroneously been stated. Markova's sister, Doris Barry, performed at the Windmill which specialised in non-stop *Revudeville* (see Chapter 3).

44 The history of the 'Ballet Russe' companies of the 1930s and later is complicated and dogged by personality clashes and ballet politics. The following is an outline. It begins with René Blum, a director at the Casino Theatre, Monte Carlo, attempting to programme ballet after Diaghilev's death. (It had been the home theatre of his company.) From 1932 this grew into a touring company jointly directed by Blum and de Basil, Les Ballets Russes de Monte Carlo. They toured some of the old Diaghilev repertory and employed the celebrated choreographers who worked with Diaghilev: Fokine, Massine, Nijinska and Balanchine. In 1938, following tension between Blum and de Basil, and the disaffection of Massine, the then resident choreographer, a rival company emerged, directed by Blum and Massine, Ballet Russe de Monte Carlo. De Basil continued with his company, later titled the Original Ballet Russe to distinguish it. Both companies suffered from the strains of constant American tours during World War II and declined in the postwar years, the Original Ballet Russe virtually ceasing in 1948, with an unsuccessful attempt at revival in 1951. The Ballet Russe de Monte Carlo, under the later management of Serge Denham, was disbanded in

1962.

45 P.W. Manchester, 'Mia Slavenska and the Polovtsian Dances from "Prince Igor"', *Ballet Today*, August 1951, p.16; Peter Williams, 'Dance and Dancers...at Home', *Dance and Dancers*, August 1951, p.19; Arnold Haskell (1952) 'Outstanding Events of the Year', *Ballet Annual, Sixth Issue*, p.36.

46 Arnold Haskell (1952) 'Outstanding Events of the Year', *Ballet Annual, Sixth Issue*, p.7.

47 'The Stoll: "Giselle"', *The Stage*, 24 May 1951, p.10.

48 'The Sitter Out', *The Dancing Times*, June 1951, pp. 514-516; Arnold Haskell (1952) 'Outstanding Events of the Year', *Ballet Annual, Sixth Issue*, p.28.

49 See Anton Dolin (1953) *Markova: Her Life and Art*, pp.225-226 for an account of the beginnings of the ballet. Markova, Danilova and Krassovska had previously appeared together in the ballet, staged for the Ballet Russe de Monte Carlo in New York, 1949.

50 Lionel Bradley thinks this after the performance of 4 June 1951. Ballet Bulletins, 4 June 1951.

51 See: Arnold Haskell (1952) 'Outstanding Events of the Year', *Ballet Annual, Sixth Issue*, p.4.

52 This description is based upon the following accounts and films: 'The Stoll: "Pas de Quatre"', *The Stage*, 7 June 1951, p.9; *The Romantic Era* (1980), ABC Video Enterprises (Alicia Alonso, Carla Fracci, GhislaineThesmar, and Eva Evdokimova); The following at NYPL Jerome Robbins Dance Division: Rehearsal of Royal Winnipeg Ballet production, filmed in April 1968 at Manitoba Centennial Concert Hall, Winnipeg (Christine Hennessy, Sheila MacKinnon, Donna Miller, and Alexandra Nadal) *MGZIC 9-4959; Excerpts from the Ballet Russe de Monte Carlo production of *Pas de quatre* filmed by Ann Barzel 'mid-1950s' (Alicia Markova, Patricia Wilde, Alexandra Danilova, Gertrude Tyven) *MGZIA 4-3605.

53 Lionel Bradley, Ballet Bulletins, 16 June 1951; *Dance and Dancers*, August 1951, p.16.

54 'Commentary', *Ballet*, January/February 1951, p.4; P.W. Manchester 'Festival Ballet at the Stoll', *Ballet Today*, January 1951, pp.4-5.

55 Part of the tunnel is now used for the Aldwych road underpass. Tram tracks can still be seen at the upper end of the tunnel in Southampton Row.

56 The Lyceum has been famed as home of the musical, *The Lion King* since 1999.

57 *Picture Post*, 30 June 1951, pp.20-23.

58 Richard Buckle, 'Commentary', *Ballet*, March 1950, p.5.

59 P.J.S. Richardson, 'Ten Year's Work: The Progress of "International Ballet"', *The Dancing Times*, July 1951, pp.583-585.

60 Sergeyev died in June 1951. Obituary: Cyril Beaumont (1952) 'Nicholas Grigorievitch Sergeyev' in Arnold Haskell, ed. (1952) *Ballet Annual, Sixth Issue*, pp.56-59.

61 For a discussion of Inglesby and her choreography see Karen Eliot (2012) 'English in Flavor and Form: Mona Inglesby's Choreography for the International Ballet', *Ballet Chronicle*, v.35, no.1, 54-83.

62 Peter Williams, 'International Ballet', *Dance and Dancers*, September 1951, p.21.

63 See Eliot, ibid.

64 V&A Theatre Museum Collection, Box 2369, South Bank Royal Festival Hall, 1951-54.

65 'Festival Hall: International Ballet', *The Stage*, 2 August 1951, p.9.

66 'The Sitter Out', *The Dancing Times*, September 1951, pp.699-700; Peter Williams, 'International Ballet', *Dance and Dancers*, September 1951, p.21; Janet Sinclair, 'International Ballet at the Festival Hall', *Ballet Today*, September 1951, p.9.

67 Frank Jackson, 'Dancing in Musicals', *Ballet Today*, September 1950, pp. 15-17; Jay

Price, 'Dancing in Musicals: 1: *Carousel*', *Dance and Dancers*, August 1950, p. 14.

68 The filmed version of *Carousel* did not use de Mille's choreography. I base my knowledge of the original dances on the video documentary, *The Dances of Carousel* (1993) in which de Mille discusses them with Gemze de Lappe, demonstrated by the Nashville Ballet. Available at Jerome Robbins Dance Division, New York Public Library for the Performing Arts.

69 See: Peter Williams, 'Opera, Ballet, and Indigestion', *Dance and Dancers*, June 1951, p.16; Joan Lawson, 'The Tales of Hoffmann', *The Dancing Times*, June 1951, pp.522-523 ; Campbell Dixon 'Film Notes: Something to Remember: 'Hoffmann' is Rich and Strange', unidentified press cutting in Monica Collingwood Collection, dated in pencil 23.4.51; Monk Gibbon (1951) *The Tales of Hoffmann*, p.95; Mary Ann Peltz 'Tales of Hoffmann', *Films in Review*, May 1951, pp.44-46; Catherine de la Rock, 'Films of the Month: The Tales of Hoffmann', *Sight and Sound*, May 1951, pp.17-18.

70 *The Stage*, 'Round the Halls', 21 June 1951, p.5; 19 July 1951, p.5; 30 August 1951, p.5; 25 October 1951, p.5; *The Stage*, 'Variety Stage', 2 August 1951, p.3; 16 August 1951, p.3; Programme available in V&A Theatre Collection, Empire Theatre File, 1949-52.

71 Janet Sinclair 'An American in Paris', *Ballet Today*, October 1951, p.10. This is the only review found that includes *both* the stage show and the film!

72 Lance Treadwell 'Kelly in Paris', *Dance and Dancers*, October 1951, p.19.

73 Some new sections were composed, and some original music dropped, moved or repeated.

74 The Blogger Maria Colina gives an analysis of the art references: http://vacheespagnole.wordpress.com/2011/11/13/1951-an-american-in-paris-art-and-vincente-minnelli/ accessed 27 October 2012.

75 This is my own definition of this motif, similar to a step performed by James Cagney in the film *Yankee Doodle Dandy* (1942).

76 Philip Hope-Wallace, 'The Current Cinema: An American in Paris', *Sight and Sound*, October-December 1951, pp.77-78.

77 Nat Karson was an artist and stage designer. He brought together programmes based around a theme, for example *Jewel Box Revue* in May, which had an Emerald Isle finale. Cine-variety was apparently instituted at the Empire 1949-52 in order to combat falling revenue. But the cost of such shows was clearly too huge to maintain in the long run. The last show was on 1 March 1952. David High (1985) *The First Hundred Years: The Story of the Empire, Leicester Square*, 64-66. For Edward Noll see: Peter Williams, 'Two moccasins to forty-eight taps', *Dance and Dancers*, January 1952, p.10.

78 Dancers in the Empire Ballet included Annette Chappell, Jeanne Artois, Brenda Hamlyn, Leo Kersley.

79 Alan Carter spoke about learning from Edward Noll's way of working. Interview with the author, 18 July 1995.

80 David Bieda of the Seven Dials Trust, responsible for erecting a facsimile column in the late 1980s, reports teenagers offering flowers and dancing around it one early morning. *BBC Home* (2008) 'London Places: The Rise and Fall ... and Rise Again of Seven Dials', : http://www.bbc.co.uk/london/content/articles/2008/09/01/seven_dials_feature.shtml, accessed 13 November 2012. [no longer available Feb 2013].

81 English Heritage gave it Grade II listing in 1999 as an early example of 'Germanic moderne [late Art Deco] forms of simple shapes enlivened by concealed lighting, shiny steelwork and touches of bright colour'. English Heritage, Cambridge Theatre entry http://list.english-heritage.org.uk/resultsingle.aspx?uid=1342096, accessed

13 November 2012.

82 The Theatres Trust, Cambridge Theatre entry, available from: http://www. theatrestrust.org.uk/resources/theatres/show/1984-cambridge-theatre-london, accessed 13 November 2012.

83 Richard Buckle (1953) *Adventures of a Ballet Critic*, p.270.

84 Elsa Brunelleschi, 'Teresa and Luisillo and their Company of Spanish Dancers', *Ballet*, May 1951, pp.49-51.

85 Elsa Brunelleschi, 'Antonio on Television', *Ballet*, April 1950, pp.41-44.

86 Richard Buckle, 'Ballet', *The Observer*, 10 September 1951, p.6.

87 Richard Buckle (1953) *The Adventures of a Ballet Critic*, pp.208, 209.

88 Ibid. p.207.

89 'From Seville to Seven Dials: Rosario and Antonio Bring Spain to London', *The Stage*, 21 June 1951, p.1; 'The Cambridge: Rosario and Antonio', *The Stage*, 28 June 1951 p.9.

90 Lionel Bradley, Ballet Bulletins, 14 June 1951.

91 Elsa Brunelleschi, 'Rosario and Antonio again', *Ballet*, January 1952, pp.21-25.

92 'The Sitter Out', *The Dancing Times*, September 1951, pp.700-701.

93 Arnold Haskell (1952) 'Outstanding Events of the Year', *Ballet Annual, Sixth Issue*, pp.47, 48.

94 Mary Clarke (1953) 'Grand Ballet du Marquis de Cuevas at the Cambridge Theatre', in Arnold Haskell, ed. *Ballet Annual, Seventh Issue*, pp.7-8.

95 Arnold Haskell (1953) 'Outstanding Events of the Year', in *Ballet Annual, Seventh Issue*, pp.8-11.

96 Arnold Haskell (1953) 'Outstanding Events of the Year', in *Ballet Annual, Seventh Issue*, pp.11-12; *The Dancing Times*, December 1951, pp.133-134.

97 See 'Schoolgirl Nonsense', *Ballet*, February 1952, pp.32,38, in which quotations from critics are compared to indicate this split, 'a Buckle-Brunelleschi-*Ballet* bloc in favour of Antonio, and a Haskell-R.A.D.-*Dancing Times* bloc in favour of Greco'.

98 Lisa Gordon-Smith 'Spain in Islington and Seven Dials', *Ballet Today*, August 1951, pp.21-23.

99 'London–Believe It or Not', *Picture Post*, 23 June 1951, unpag.

100 Frank Jackson, 'Editorial Comment', *Ballet Today*, December 1951, p.3.

101 Peter Williams, [untitled editorial], *Dance and Dancers*, August 1951, p.4.

102 Richard Buckle, 'Commentary', *Ballet*, July 1952, p.5.

CHAPTER THREE

1952: TOO MUCH BALLET!

January
26th : A state of emergency is declared after rioting against British troops in the Suez Canal Zone, Egypt. Deaths in Ismailia and Cairo.

February
6th : Death of King George VI at Sandringham , the royal estate in Norfolk.

On 11 February three queens attend as the body of the late King is taken from Sandringham Church to Westminster Hall in London: Queen Elizabeth II, Queen Elizabeth the Queen Mother, and the Dowager Queen Mary. They are dressed in black, their faces hardly seen beneath the black gauze veils that cover them to the waist. Between them they span a period that reaches back into the reign of Queen Victoria. Unlike the other queens, Queen Mary, upright and indomitable, is dressed to the ankle in her still Edwardian fashion. Instead of her more usual toque she wears a close-fitting, black cap coming to a sharp V on her forehead, a version of mourning headwear introduced at the death of Queen Victoria.[1] The train arrives at King's Cross and the procession proceeds along Euston Road, receiving the acknowledgement of dignitaries and people. Near Euston Station it turns south along a route that takes it past the Stoll Theatre in Kingsway, through Aldwych and the Strand to Whitehall. The *Ars Magna* of London takes to the streets once more. On this occasion, though, there is something more than the draw of ritual performed to its most exquisite level. The King represents survival, the coming-through of the wartime experience. During the days of lying-in-state in Westminster Hall doors must be kept open for the queues of people to file past until 2 am and then on the final night until 6 am.

The coffin moves through London again on 15 February, to be buried at Windsor in St George's Chapel. The sound track of the day is of minute guns, maroons, the tolling bell of Big Ben; the tramp of boots as the naval ratings haul the gun carriage; barked orders, pipes and drums. Then, at 2pm, the two minutes of silence. The Lord Chamberlain has ordered theatres to be closed until 6 pm as a mark of respect, so the evening performances can go ahead.

*   *   *   *   *

The dance year has begun with a controversy which blows up in the press, questioning the very worth of ballet, the intelligence of its adherents, and the competence of its critics. On the anti-ballet side are theatre producer Tyrone Guthrie, theatre critic Alan Dent, and grumpy television personality

Gilbert Harding. In the opposite corner are ballet critics including Richard Buckle and Arnold Haskell. As a fan, Monica is aware of the fuss, preserving Dent's article in her scrapbook. Guthrie begins the debate in the pages of *News Chronicle*, with the view that ballet has nothing new to offer. Musical theatre is the coming thing. 'In five years we'll have OUR 'Oklahoma'... In ten years light opera will be the dominant form of theatrical expression'.[2] So Guthrie denies the power of dance, without words, to communicate anything. Dent as *News Chronicle* theatre critic then weighs in with some considerable slurs against ballet-goers:

> Grown-ups who are too fond of ballet become pampered, fractious, and silly, like children who have access to too many sweets and ices. The regular and insatiable supporters of ballet are people too sluggish of intellect to listen to a play on the one hand, and too devoid of imagination to listen to fine music without accompanying action, on the other.[3]

And he finds ballet critics 'humourless and intense', quoting Buckle's public reply to Guthrie in *The Observer* as evidence. (Buckle did in fact lay on rather thickly the benefits of ballet-viewing on the 'soul' of the spectator.)[4]

Considering that the main antagonists are critics, surely more clarity of argument could be expected on both sides. The central 'anti' arguments are ones with which many ballet critics concur (as they have been telling us for some time!): there is not enough good, new choreography; the constant revivals of nineteenth century ballets clog the repertoire; ballet fans are obsessed with stars and uncritical of performance.[5] So where does this attack come from? It's not difficult to see that some jealousy is involved. Guthrie directs operas as well as plays, and was the overall head of the Old Vic and Sadler's Wells Theatres (1939-1945) after the death of Lilian Baylis. The Sadler's Wells Ballet was taken out of his control and given its high altar at the Royal Opera House, while opera struggled to find its authentic Covent Garden 'voice'.[6] Consequently ballet has enjoyed a fulsome press up to now, with the glamour of its female stars and tours to North America from which the country earns some much needed revenue. When they go abroad the dancers are provided with clothing and accessories from British manufacturers to model. Fashion loves the ballet physique. Those tiny waists and long legs suit the latest female fashions: the 'tailored look' with the tight waist and long pencil skirt, or the 'ballerina length' dress flaring out in a wide skirt from its tight belt. There are hair styles and decorations apparently inspired by 'the craze for ballet'.[7] Even television is taking ballet seriously! Since 1949 there have been twenty ballet performances on the only television channel quite apart from the educational *Ballet for Beginners* series. There is even a Television Ballet Group on contract. Covent Garden

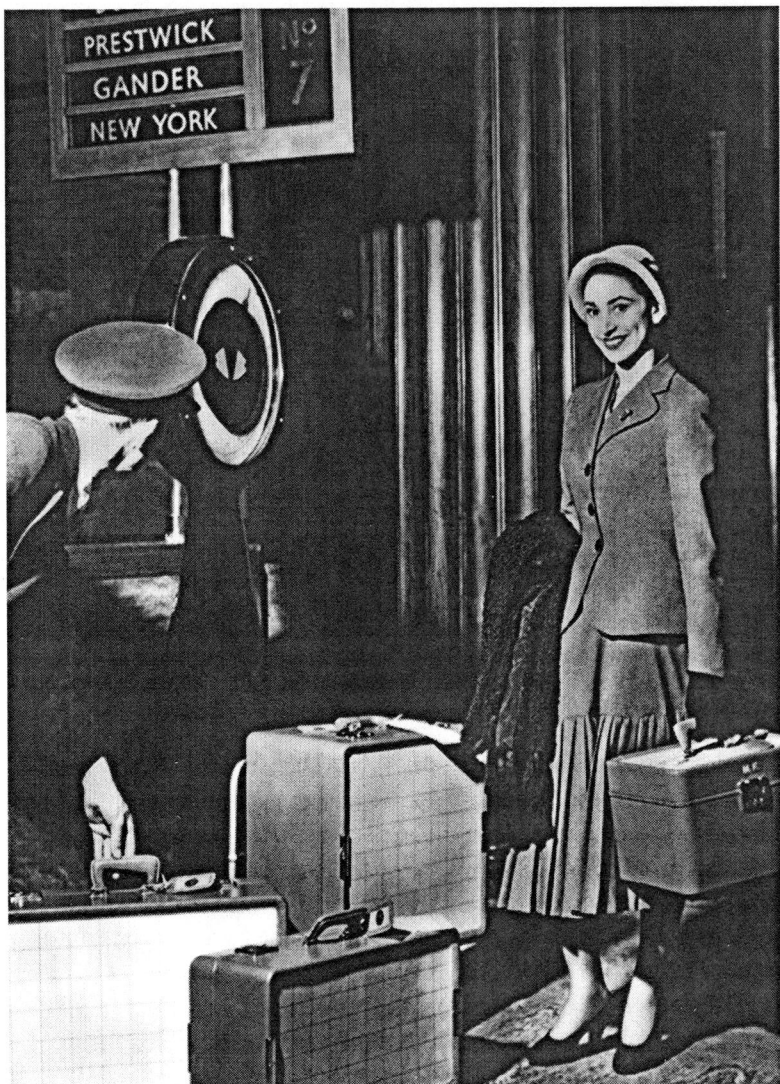

Margot Fonteyn at the BOAC terminal, London, bound for a tour of the USA and Canada with travel goods manufactured for her by Papworth Industries at Cambridge.
Photo: © Keystone /Getty Images.

now takes the lion's share of the Arts Council subsidy, yet the foundation stone for a National Theatre for play production in London, laid on the South Bank during the Festival of Britain, is not materialising.[8]

Perhaps getting to the crux of the matter is the anonymous writer of the 'Pendennis' column in *The Observer*, who rather more calmly notes that ballet was put on a pedestal directly after the war, becoming 'a national sacred cow'. But now there are 'cracks in the pedestal' because that reputation depends upon stars like Shearer (famous from the films *The Red Shoes* and

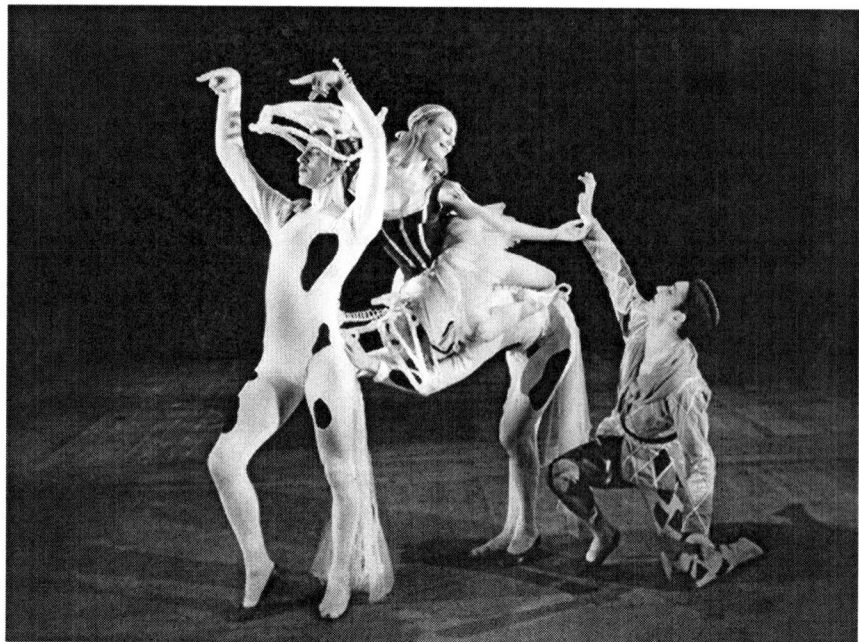

Antoinette Sibley, as Columbine riding a unicorn, and David Blair as Harlequin, in *Harlequin in April* (chor. Cranko, 1951). This photo by G.B.L. Wilson is from the 1959 production at Covent Garden. © Royal Academy of Dance/ArenaPAL.

Tales of Hoffmann) and Fonteyn in the old classical works. Clearly this cannot be maintained.[9] It always makes good 'copy' to tear down a pedestal, to humble the over-confident, and make the less fortunate feel better.

In decrying ballet's staid image, I suspect that Guthrie, Dent and Pendennis did not see any of the new works from 1951 that were extending the art form in new directions, to take two admired by Lionel Bradley, Cranko's *Harlequin in April* at Sadler's Wells and Ashton's *Tiresias* at Covent Garden. Both of these won Arts Council grants to cover new music compositions (from Richard Arnell and Constant Lambert respectively) for the Festival of Britain Season.[10] Neither dealt with fairy stories of conventional love. None of the trappings of ballet that are supposed to 'pamper' the audience with too much sweetness were in evidence and they certainly contained enough allegory and allusions to test the intellect of the spectator. In Cranko's complex story Harlequin is born out of the earth and returns to it after a dalliance with a dishevelled Columbine who may also be a plant. Pierrot and a whole herd of unicorns help and hinder him. In *Tiresias* the male Tiresias is turned into a female Tiresias for the act of striking two copulating snakes and then turned back again for repeating this act. He is struck blind by the goddess Hera when, having experienced both, he agrees with Zeus that women get more pleasure than men in sex. To say this ballet caused a scandal would be putting it mildly, not just because of the subject matter but because it was over-long. However, we have not seen the last of it and it comes back into the repertoire in a shortened form this year of 1952.

February
21st : Wartime identity cards abolished.

March
17th : Utility clothing scheme ends.
27th : Cheese ration reduced to one ounce (28 grams) per week.

May
2nd : First scheduled air liner, BOAC Comet, Heathrow to Johannesburg, takes off.

From Covent Garden to the South Bank

Covent Garden is an eccentric combination of commerce and culture. The streets are all about the common-or-garden daily necessity of food for the capital and the daily necessity of physical labour to provide it. It is in fact a fully functioning wholesale market where the sacks and boxes of fruit, vegetables and flowers are auctioned and sold on. The people of the market are regular Londoners, shabby but implacable in their centuries of tradition. Porters zealously guard their privileges to load and unload, hauling stuff around in wooden barrows and carried on their heads. (They have an annual competition for the highest basket tower a porter can run with!) There are flower sellers, much like Eliza in George Bernard Shaw's *Pygmalion* (1912) and women sit shelling peas. Incongruously, all this takes place in the seventeenth century Italianate Piazza by Inigo Jones. The portico of Jones's St Paul's Church shelters market people and theatre goers just as in *Pygmalion*. The contours of roofed halls, columns, porticos and colonnades in the nineteenth century neo-classical style hardly seem to emerge from the obscurity of the piles and stacks. The domed glass and iron Floral Hall, looking so much like a miniature Crystal Palace, is the foreign fruit market.[11] Lorries clog the streets to the market area. It's a loud, bustling, irreverent place; yet, all of this encircles a supposed ivory tower of high culture. At the eastern end of the Piazza is the 1858 Royal Opera House, third on this site. Here, even in 1952, audiences of the stalls and circle are often in evening dress and, on gala nights, it is *de rigeur*. By the evening the market has cleared away, to start up again soon after the last of the performers and staff have left the Nag's Head pub near the Opera House stage door.[12]

Commerce and culture were brought together literally on the ground in the completion of purchase of this estate, including the market and Opera House, in 1918. The new owner, buying from the Dukes of Bedford, was the family pharmaceutical company, famous for its Beecham's Pills. Sir Joseph

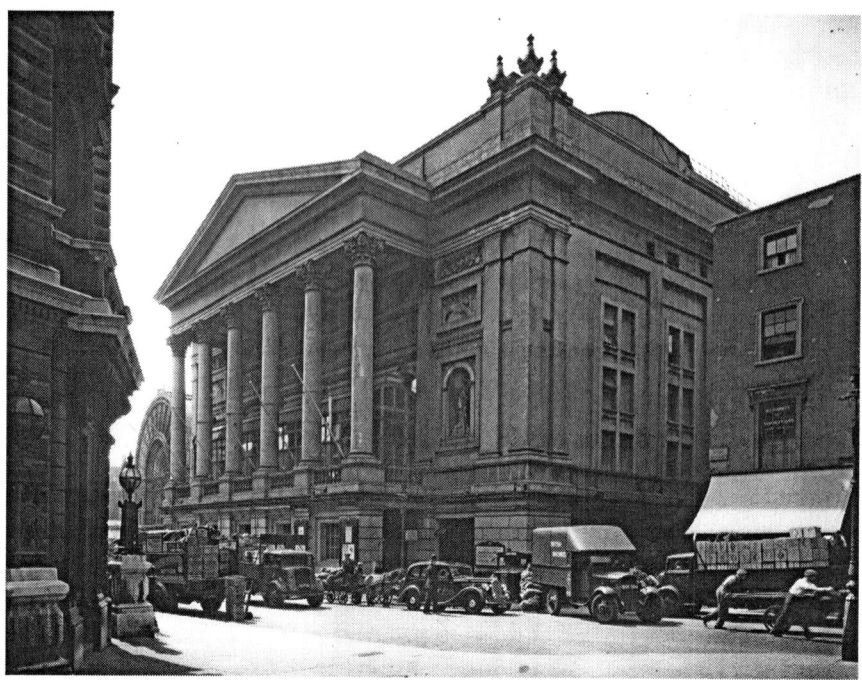

The Royal Opera House, Covent Garden, in 1948, including market traffic, Floral Hall in the distance and the entrance to Bow Street Magistrates Court in the left foreground. The notice on the Opera House wall advertises the Marquis de Cuevas, Grand Ballet de Monte Carlo which performed there during August. Photo: © Topical Press Agency/ Getty Images.

Beecham and his conductor son, Sir Thomas Beecham, were supporters and impresarios for Diaghilev before World War I. (Commerce and culture again!) Diaghilev's company gave its final London season at Covent Garden in 1929, and there were seasons of Colonel de Basil's Ballets Russes here in the 1930s, giving some help to Sir Thomas's opera seasons, while the future of the House was often under threat from 'redevelopment'. Now in 1952, those problems for a continued life for the Opera House are behind us and Sir Thomas was praised last year for his conducting of the film of *The Tales of Hoffmann*. With the benefit of a sizeable subsidy from the Arts Council of Great Britain, this has become the nation's principal establishment for ballet and opera.[13] The Royal Opera House lives up to its name as the site of galas for visiting royal and state dignitaries.

The Opera House and the Floral Hall show their imposing frontages on Bow Street, facing the Police Station and Magistrates' Court. Here is another long historical tradition of Covent Garden. To commerce and culture we must add law and order. There has been a seat of law in various locations along Bow Street for centuries. Henry Fielding, novelist of that picaresque tale of a country youth in London, *Tom Jones* (1749), presided here as magistrate in the eighteenth century and instituted his band of 'Bow Street Runners' to apprehend criminals.[14]

Anatole Chujoy, editor of the US publication *Dance News*, thinks very highly of the Opera House interior compared to other great opera houses of the world. It's intimate in scale, so it's easy to make friends here, and while the leg room is rather restricted, other comforts are on offer in the bars and snacks at each level and even tea and ice-cream in the auditorium during intervals. What is more, he thinks rather more highly of the ballet audience here than do Alan Dent and some of our ballet critics. He *does* find the Covent Garden audiences discerning and more open-minded than most of the press![15]

July
5th : Last London trams run.
26th : King Farouk of Egypt forced to abdicate by a coup of army officers including Colonel Nasser and General Naguib .

August
19th : Lynmouth, N. Devon, flood disaster kills over 30.
20th : State of emergency declared in Kenya after growing unrest and attacks from Mau Mau guerrillas.

New York City Ballet takes up residence at the Royal Opera House, Covent Garden, from 7 July for six weeks. This is guaranteed to ruffle some feathers. The previous visit of 1950 succeeded in dividing opinion. As much as it's good to have them visit London again in 1952 (it is, after all, 'the dance capital of the world'), George Balanchine's young company seems to rewrite all the rules. Balanchine has dared to choreograph his own version of *Swan Lake Act II* and of the beloved Diaghilev/Fokine ballet, *The Firebird*. (It was a real mistake to programme this on the opening night).[16] He's also making dances that rely totally on choreography and music, without plot or décor to help the viewer. His *Ballet Imperial*, is performed by our own Sadler's Wells Ballet, but too much plotless work on a programme can be tedious especially when the décors are plain. Caryl Brahms, apt and witty as ever, blames Balanchine, 'for being the worst programme-builder that ever defeated the natural high spirits of the dancer and the danced-to.' The visual austerity of 'white tunic, or tu-tu, against a black curtain, black tunic or tu-tu, against white cyclorama' etc., defeats her concentration if it happens too often on a programme, despite the sometimes brilliance of the choreographic invention. 'I blame Balanchine for putting me to the misery of being unable to respond.'[17] The Diaghilev model of a ballet, one which has been received wisdom for decades, makes theme and design as essential to the artistic expression as choreography and music. It would be wrong to suggest that the plotless kind of ballet is the only thing he can do. American critic Edwin Denby lists Balanchine's ballet types as: 'dance ballet, drama with plot, drama of atmosphere, comedy of situation...exhibition pas de deux'.[18] He brings his *Orpheus* to London, for example, and the revival of his *Prodigal Son* from Diaghilev days but the heart of the repertoire seems to rest in his demanding, stripped-down 'dance ballet' vocabulary in spite of the markedly different contributions of his other choreographers, William Dollar, Ruthanna Boris, Jerome Robbins and Antony Tudor. Monica attends only twice during the season and writes no comment, so it appears she is not enthusiastic. (Contrastingly, in June she made seven visits to the Opera House or Sadler's Wells for the 'home' companies.) Richard Buckle leads the charge in favour of Balanchine and the New York City Ballet, with large parts of the July, August and September editions of *Ballet* devoted to them. For him, Balanchine is 'the greatest choreographer of our day'.[19]

There are some pieces that could just be in bad taste – take Jerome Robbins's *The Cage*, with female dancers imitating predatory insects, killing their mates after sex. There is a suggestion of a web in the decor of strings and wavy lines on the females' beige leotards. But what we see initially is a female cult, with a Queen and a 'Novice'. This is a bit like *Giselle* Act II except that the Novice has no intention of saving any of her male victims. She is the willing convert to the cult, testing her strength then rising to the occasion. She uses her arms like pincers and striates one against the other. The first male intruder gets the full stamping, throwing and neck-breaking between her thighs. The second male intruder is rather more beguiling, more pressing in his advances and less easy to throw off. They curve their bodies deeply towards each other, pelvises forward in sexual excitement. Sacrifice is achieved by the full attack of the cult. There really is something ugly and repugnant here.[20] Is it appropriate on a ballet stage? Caryl Brahms thinks it 'aesthetically as pleasing as a guttersnipe who chalks a rude work up in the Loo'.[21] Perhaps the visual vulnerability of the men is also quite unnerving, stripped of everything but what appears to be half a loin cloth, bare legged, shoeless and apparently with one bare hip. *Picture Post* declares: 'Broadway hailed it. Paris raved about it. But London audiences find 'The Cage' just a rather dreary and unpleasant episode in the otherwise fine programme...' It is 'degrading' and 'ingeniously nasty' but presumably not so degrading and nasty as all that, because the magazine makes fully sensationalist use of the photographs.[22]

Or is it breaking new ground? After three viewings, Lionel Bradley decides that he does not like this 'stark, exciting work', but it seems to be a perfect realisation of the Stravinsky music.[23] Contrast this with his strong reaction against Balanchine's stripped-down, plotless *Concerto Barocco*, 'mechanical' to the point of being 'nauseating'.[24]

Few would deny that Balanchine's choreography is intriguing, and that he has an array of worthy ballerinas of different personalities (the men are a

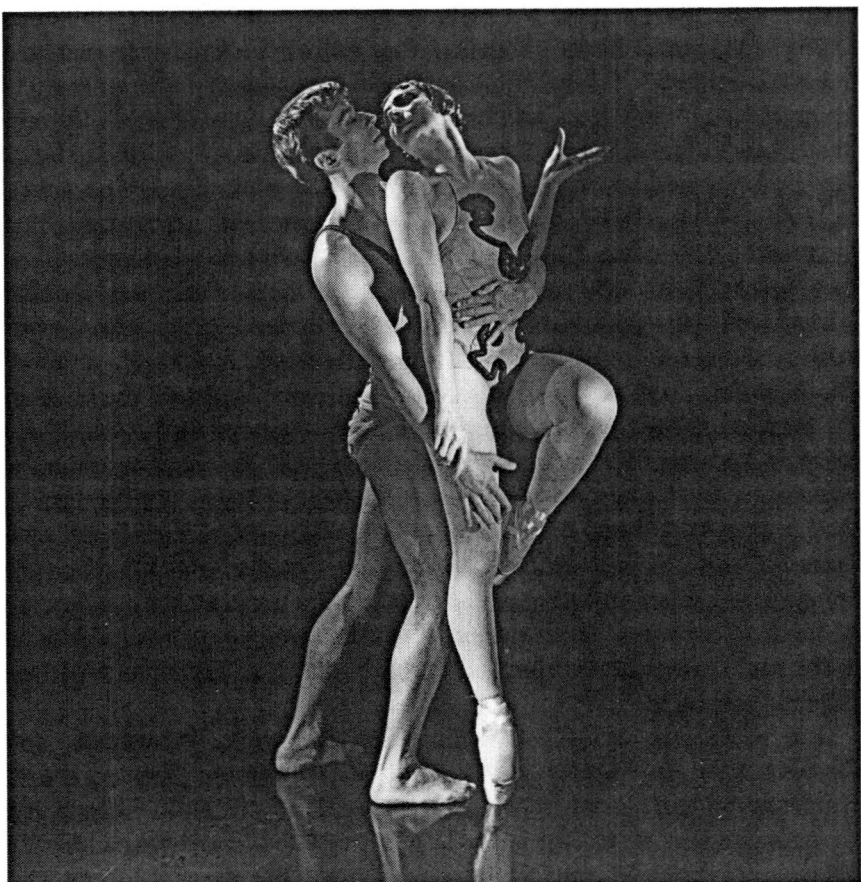

Nora Kaye and Nicholas Magallanes of New York City Ballet in *The Cage* (chor. Robbins, 1951). Photo: © Baron/Getty Images.

bit lacking in interest). But his plotless choreography is taxing to the viewer. It appears that we prefer the Americana pieces. This is what we expect from a company from across the water.[25] Fun is something much easier to understand than formalism. *The Pied Piper* is set by Jerome Robbins to Aaron Copland's *Clarinet Concerto*, a jazzy piece, typically American, we assume. The clarinet makes the dancers do silly things, jive and generally be young and uncontrolled. *Cakewalk* by Ruthanna Boris pretends to take place on a Mississippi showboat with acts performed to popular tunes.[26]

On first encountering *The Four Temperaments*, some of us are inclined to mutter, 'oh no, it's one of those', (plotless, practice dress pieces).[27] It was presented in 1950 with dreadful costumes, now it has been stripped back to leotards, tights and t-shirts, so it seems we are being forced to see the music (by Hindemith[28]) and hear the dance. But what is it saying? Is this a commentary on the classical style? It begins with three *pas de deux* that

seem to raise this question. The first one starts formally with the gentleman
offering his hand to his lady. Together, they make a few extensions of legs, a
few *ronds de jambes*. This is tantalisingly like the classical dance we seem to
know, although they seem cold towards each other. A *pas de deux* is usually
about love, but these people don't seem to know it. Then they start to break
down all the certainties of ballet technique. She walks forward on *pointe*,
but flexing the foot before she puts it down; *pirouettes* with a bent supporting
knee; sticks her extended leg *between* his, which looks a little indecent. When
he manhandles her offstage, trying to look as if she is in one long leap that
never touches the ground, we realise that he has never let go of her for one
minute. The second *pas de deux*, with a different couple, is more dynamic and
playful but again there is a sense that the technique and even the limits of
the body are being tested by manipulation. At one point he has her by the
waist and promenades her around, pressing out her hips one way, then the
other. Hips don't usually move this way in classical ballet. The third *pas de
deux* is more lyrical and there's a lot of wrapping around each other, with
arms and legs. Again there's a variation of the classical tradition when the
ballerina is paddled around in *pirouette* by tapping her extended arm instead
of turning her waist. There seems to be something emotionally detached
in the performance, as if to imply that this is all just an experiment into the
physically possible.

The variations are called Melancholic, Sanguinic, Phlegmatic, and
Choleric, after the ancient theory of the four humours dictating mood,
temperament and health. In each there is a central solo or duet expressing
the temperament, then being joined by a group of dancers who exemplify the
opposite or become infected by the central mood. There is more drama and
wit here. The male solo in Melancholic is always striving and falling. Some
of the girls that come to support him seem to copy his depression at times,
weighted down by the effort. In Phlegmatic there are movement motifs that
look like sighs and shrugs. In Choleric there are bursts of impatience as
dancers pull each other to new locations but it ends on an optimistic note
with a full cast finale, the company in lines, and the principal women being
borne up by their partners in high leaps crossing the stage.[29]

So the ending of *The Four Temperaments* sounds and looks rather noble
and inspiring. Perhaps the choreography has been more about the formal
qualities of theme and variations than about the temperaments. Clever
reiterations of recognised motifs keep recurring: the jutting hips, the flexed
ankles, traceries of arms and legs, certain kinds of lifts. These are 'dance
jokes' for the initiated but in themselves they also seem to ask questions.
What is the future for classical ballet? Does it go on evolving by breaking its
own technical rules of how to do a *pirouette*, or where to place the foot, or
what the hips should do? Do we see this as destructive of cherished values

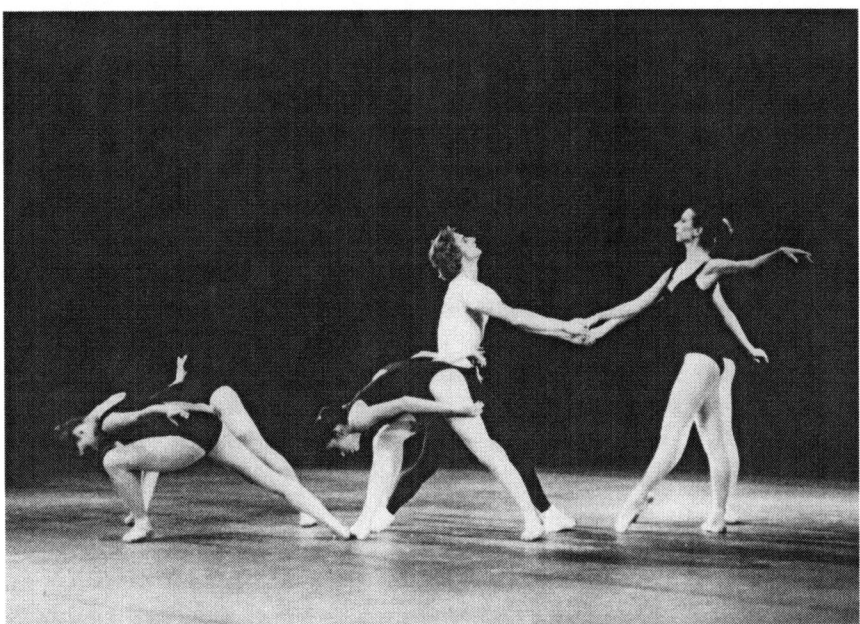

Bart Cook, Delia Peters and New York City Ballet performing in 1977 'Melancholic' from *The Four Temperaments* (chor. Balanchine, 1946). No photographer credit. Jerome Robbins Dance Division, the New York Public Library for the Performing Arts, Astor, Lenox and Tilden Foundations.

or, like Edwin Denby, as a new kind of classicism and a limitless source of beautiful images based in structure?[30]

*   *   *   *   *

These questions can be mulled over on the short walk to the Royal Festival Hall. Crossing Waterloo Bridge, the weather is fine for once, and there is the absolute wonder of the open skyline and the view from St Paul's to Big Ben. Between Covent Garden and the South Bank the contrasts are massive but in some ways parallel. Covent Garden is the seat of centuries of tradition, currently housing a form of ballet that seems intent on pushing tradition into the background. Over on the South Bank, the modernist Festival Hall is presenting a ballet company whose repertoire is steeped in the traditions of the nineteenth and early twentieth centuries. The environment of each theatre is chaotic in its own way, the Opera House in its usual marketplace way and the Festival Hall now standing amidst the deconstructed ruins of what was the South Bank Exhibition of last year. The jumbled remains of exhibits have been seen in a builder's yard in Gospel Oak, North London.[31]

Festival Ballet (now titling itself 'London's Festival Ballet') has its season here for the first time from 31 July, overlapping with the New York City Ballet, so some enthusiasts like Lionel Bradley are alternating their attendances north and south of the river. Considering what a disaster the Royal Festival Hall has been as a venue for ballet so far, it is surprising that Festival Ballet want to quit the Stoll for this place. There must have been soul searching. What are the factors? Against the move is the set-up of the auditorium and backstage from the company's point of view but if these can be surmounted, the audience gets superb facilities. The company's stage director, Ben Toff, has transformed the stage into a proscenium using steel tubing and draperies. Flying of scenery is not possible but for some ballets they can project backcloth designs onto a high quality cyclorama, while for others backcloths must be taken down and rolled at each interval.[32] Later in the season it looks as if the projections are proving ineffective.[33] These problems will be solved in time as regular ballet seasons have been announced for Festival Hall. It looks as if London's Festival Ballet has found a London home and a regular summer season here will be to ballet what the Promenade Concerts (Proms) at the Albert Hall are to music, that is to say, a venue that favours a popular and youthful audience.[34]

The venue is not the only problem, since Markova has left the company, initially with a foot injury, leaving Nathalie Krassovska (now Nathalie Leslie, using the surname of her Russo-Scottish father, rather than her mother's Russian name) as prima ballerina. On opening night Dolin's curtain speech proves controversial.

> We have no psychological ballets in our repertoire...nor do I, as artistic director of the company, intend to present ballets depicting the sordid side of life...ballets which, in my opinion, are best left in the kitchen sink.

His comments are assumed to be directed at the repertoire of the New York City Ballet, particular at Jerome Robbins's *The Cage*, although he hotly denies that he would be so ill-mannered. Yet he cannot resist labouring the point that there is a deplorable trend in ballet towards 'an unhealthy concentration on rather dreary sex'.

> I shall always protest against anything and everything which in my opinion debases our gracious and lovely art. I do not think that vulgarity and near obscenity which the good old Music Hall would never have countenanced have any place in the ballet.[35]

Well, so much for extending the boundaries of the art form! But on 1 September, they present a successful new work, perfectly in tune with the surroundings of the Festival Hall. *Symphony for Fun* is choreographed by Michael Charnley, who was previously a dancer with the modern dance company Ballets Jooss and in commercial theatre in America. He has been having some success in putting on small pieces at Ballet Workshop,

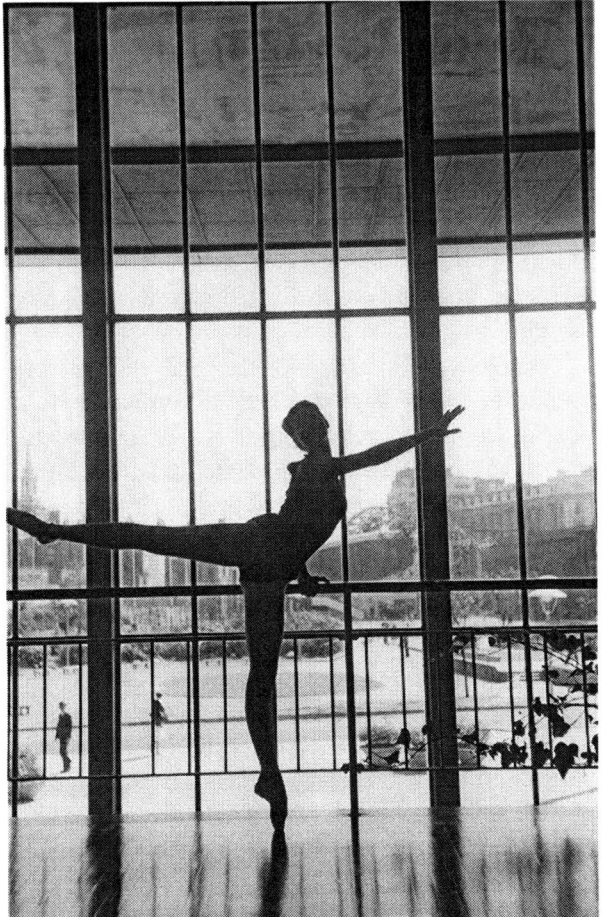

Daphne Dale of London's Festival Ballet dancing on a landing inside the Royal Festival Hall, 1953. This view towards Waterloo was obscured by subsequent building up of the area. Photo: ©John Chillingworth/Getty Images.

the choreographic platform run by Ballet Rambert and one of those, *Movimientos*, is now in the repertoire of Ballet Rambert.

The back of the stage is made to look rather like a vast window, with a low wall topped by a slatted screen resembling Venetian blinds.[36] The dancers behind the blinds are seen in silhouette. They enter in pairs each with individual motifs, in bright costumes that seem stylish and youthful. The women all have dresses with swinging, flared skirts, lined with a contrasting colour that flashes as they dance. The men have tunics that open to the waist with broad collar facings in white. Their trousers are the knee length 'pedal pushers' that have become fashionable wear.[37] The sixteen dancers are in four colour groups, women in pink and green, and men in yellow and blue. Within each group there are four shades of the colour, so the whole scene is vibrant. The first two couples are in the green/yellow combination of colours, the second two in the pink/blue combination, and this pattern is repeated.

The music conveys a good-natured mood of rivalry, high spirits and rhythmic urgency. There is one theme that has an invigorating, dotted, galloping rhythm which has a hint of the prairie about it and a clarinet solo with jazz inflections. The music is *Symphony no. 5½* by American composer, Don Gillis, so there is some reason to find some American references here.[38] Dancers perform different duet sections, some of which are watched by other dancers seated in a semi-circle. Each duet is a cameo of a relationship. A girl squeals with delight as she is lifted; a boy and girl are tongue-tied in each other's presence; a girl brushes off her boyfriend's advances.

The next movement, titled 'Scherzophrenia' seems almost 'schizophrenic' musically in a mixed bag of references to different musical genres – the Scherzo from Mendelssohn's *A Midsummer Night's Dream*, jazz, Gershwin-like street bustling music, rumba, swing band and burlesque. In this movement coloured light effects are played on the Venetian blinds. The female soloist Noel Rossana, in a white dress, her skirt lined in black, dances with the four men in shades of blue. She mimes putting on make-up and flirts with them. Finally, the girlfriends dressed in pink drag the boys away.

The lights dim for the section called 'Spiritual?', and clouds scud across the Venetian blinds. Musically it takes an air that sounds as if it's from the American South (hence 'spiritual') for a soulful *pas de deux* of young love. John Gilpin, the male principal in black and white, makes his first appearance here dancing with Anita Landa who has a grey dress lined in pink. They are accompanied by four women who just sit and watch them, covered in lacy black shawls. The dance is steeped in yearning, a solemn moment but one that does not last too long.

The finale is 'Perpetual Emotion', fast and furious activity, a pun on *perpetuum mobile* it would seem. With hints of variety theatre and film music, there is a sense of continuously being moved on by the sounds and dance. Landa is the centre of attention for the men now. Three men leap up to her and kneel in a line. She drops a rubber ball on their heads in turn. Rossana is the centre of attention for Gilpin. For the first time they dance together, being the couple with the black/white costume contrasts. The whole cast criss-crosses the stage. They go upstage to downstage with steps and claps, and across the stage with leaps. Everyone except Landa executes a fall on a downstage diagonal, and she is left with her ball. She bounces it once, and then taps it up with the palm of her hand. Curtain!

This piece is hugely popular with audiences. The style is eclectic. There is a 'Latin American' sensuousness in mobile torso, shoulder shaking, and hip rotations. Balletic movements are modified with straight arm designs rather than rounded; multiple pirouettes are performed with the knee in

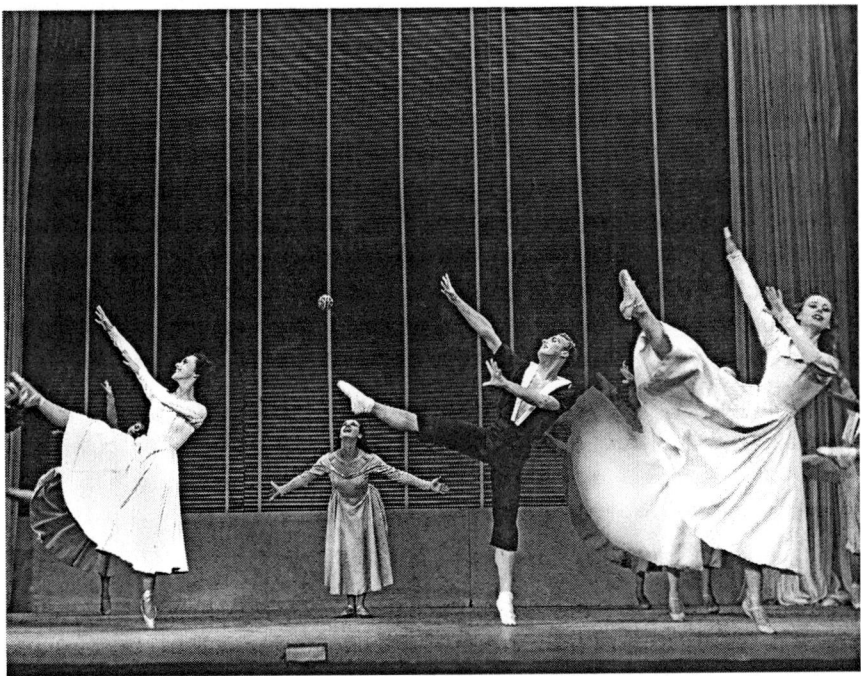

Festival Ballet in *Symphony for Fun* (chor. Charnley, 1952). Left to right: Noel Rossana, Anita Landa, John Gilpin. Photo: © Roy Round.

parallel; and only Rossana's role is choreographed for *pointe* work, with all the other dancers, including women, in soft shoes. This is quite a break with balletic tradition. Above all it is witty, sometimes in a naive way. Each time that Landa bounces the ball on the head of one of the men (in 'Perpetual Emotion'), she turns a small circle, with childish flat-footed steps. After the third head is bounced upon, she performs a kind of resigned 'shrug' with head and shoulders bending sideways, and legs bending at the knees in a turned out position, with heels coming off the floor. The men answer with the same movement and trot away from her with the same combination of turned out bent knees, on half toes.[39] It's ungainly but also endearing.

How well this fits with the company settling into its new venue! Venetian blinds on a huge window seems so 'Festival style' as is that wonderful optimism of a young company. The costumes look youthful and are worn by the youngest members of the company who have also had their hair cut short in the most fashionable style.[40] While the quirky humour – the fun with a rubber ball, the harmless flirtation – provide rather an idealised and unrealistic picture of youth, the feature of the choreography which is most true to the nature of youth is its almost constant activity. Will it still be around in fifty years' time, presenting 'a clear picture of the teenagers of 1952', as one critic believes?[41]

So Dolin appears to have succeeded in countering the complaints that the Festival Ballet repertoire is backward looking and the newer works are unsuccessful. He has done this without tapping the suggestive, erotic vein he seems to detest. *Symphony for Fun* appeals to the new audience that associates the Festival Hall with the inclusiveness of the South Bank Exhibition. In style it is somewhat similar to American musical theatre choreography and some of the lighter works of the American ballet companies, for example *Interplay* by Jerome Robbins currently being performed by the New York City Ballet. But by going down this route, is Dolin lowering the taste threshold of his audience? For *The Dancing Times* this is 'good entertainment for an unsophisticated audience'. (That puts us in our place!)

> But it is not a work to be taken seriously and coming into a repertoire composed of masterpieces by Fokine [it was premiered with *Les Sylphides* and *Petrushka*], one fears for the effect its jerky and meaningless gestures may have on the dancers' technique...[42]

* * * * *

At some point over the summer we must make a trip to Battersea Park, to the site of the splendours of the Pleasure Gardens of last year. Here, the Pleasure Gardens have reopened for the summer and the lovely little Riverside Theatre now houses an interesting experiment – 3D films. In a season of shorts, *The Black Swan* is a ballet film with a difference. What distinguishes this from the ballet programmes now becoming a regular feature on television and for the big screen is its intent to solve the technical problems of filming ballet while making the most of its movement expression. This is an attempt to access the story of *Swan Lake* through the third act Black Swan *pas de deux*. The narrative introduction (with voiceover) shows Siegfried's friend Benno returning to a ruined castle, finding a swan's feather, and remembering the subterfuge by which the Black Swan, Odile, with her magician father, Von Rothbart, deceived Prince Siegfried into believing that he was in fact dancing with the White Swan, Odette. So this plot is made to condense the spirit of the ballet into twelve minutes, with just the characters of Benno, Siegfried, Odile, Rothbart and the vision of Odette.

3D films would seem to be the coming thing. Some other shorts were produced for the Festival of Britain and have been seen in the Telecinema (originally named the Telekinema for the Exhibition) still functioning on the South Bank.[43] We have to wear cardboard glasses, with one green and one red lens. The effect is that the action seems to come towards us, out of the screen instead of on it. As an experiment this must be counted as worthwhile but it is debateable whether it has any chance of setting up a trend. The film is in black and white which seems disappointing and the scenery of swags and curtains looks flimsy, not a believable castle at all. To get the 3D effects of distance the camera often has one of the dancers in close up so that it really needs dancers with fine acting as well. Beryl Grey is perfectly seductive and David Paltenghi makes a thoroughly believable Rothbart. (A good camera trick shows his owl face change to human.) Unfortunately John Field as Siegfried is rather wooden. He doesn't seem to be totally enamoured of Odile, and therefore the plot is lost. To get its 3D effects the filming makes great use of depth. There is a long corridor for the entry and retreat of Odile and Rothbart (but those swaying drapes as they pass spoil the effect!) A row of flags is raised one by one as if the spectator is walking through the set to find Odile beginning her first variation. We often see the characters in a dramatically retreating perspective. When the vision of Odette appears at the window Rothbart is near to it, trying to hide it from Siegfried who is in the foreground with Odile near and slightly behind him. In the coda, as Siegfried finishes his pirouettes, Odile begins her *fouettés* behind him.[44] This has been an interesting experience, a new way of looking at ballet but it can't replace the genuine three dimensions of a stage performance!

West, to a real and imagined Kensington

John Cranko gets his first chance at choreographing for the main company at Covent Garden and chooses to return to the comedy genre of *Pineapple Poll*. The new ballet, *Bonne-Bouche*, is literally a tasty snack, and a satire of upper middle-class manners set amongst the classically porticoed dwellings of a recognisable South Kensington. As with *Pineapple Poll*, the sets are by the cartoonist Osbert Lancaster who is also known for drawings satirising architectural styles.[45] *Bonne-Bouche* is set in a square in Kensington, prosperous dwellings on both sides in 'Kensington Italianate' style and a mock gothic church in the background. We feel we understand what kind of people live here and some of the audience very likely do! Perhaps to avoid any ill-feeling amongst these better heeled spectators, the time period is set safely back in the Edwardian era. There is a gold-digging Mother and Daughter, a lecherous Rich Old Neighbour and others who are arty, or sporty, or theatrical 'luvvies'. Despite the period difference, these are still recognisable Kensington types, especially to high society people who are 'trained to enjoy laughing at themselves'.[46] Always on the look-out for a better prospect, the Daughter is engaged first to her Lover, then to the Rich Old Neighbour who dies from over excitement on the way to the church. Back with her original suitor, she can't resist flirting with an army officer. Totally disillusioned with her, the Lover joins a band from the League of Light and goes off to Africa to be a missionary. The drop-curtain between the scenes shows a view of Kensington Gardens and statuary around the Albert Memorial.

In a brightly painted jungle scene in the manner of Henri Rousseau, the members of the band are picked off one by one, by animals or cannibals.

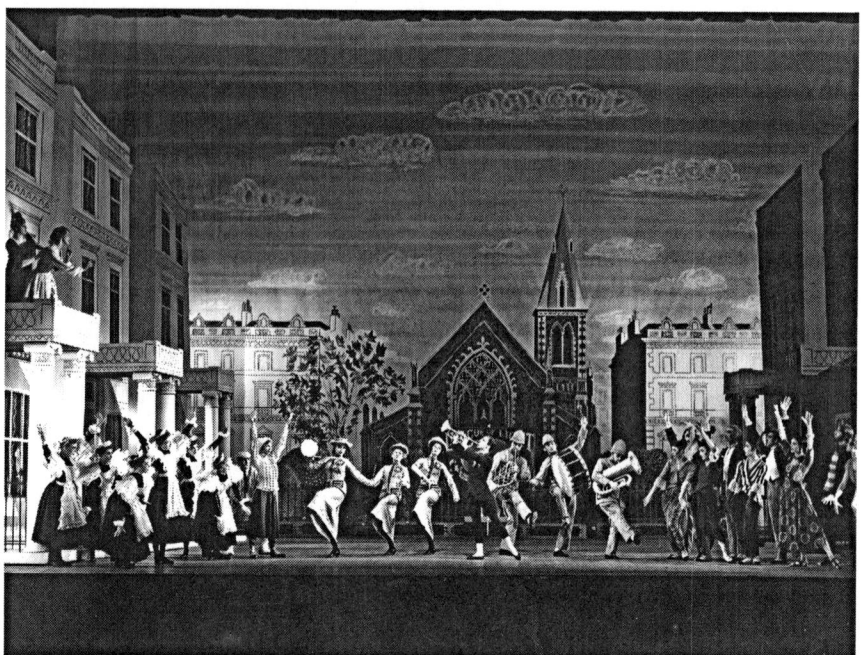

Sadler's Wells Ballet in *Bonne-Bouche* (chor. Cranko, 1952), Scene 1, a square in South Kensington (des. Osbert Lancaster), with the League of Light (centre), the Mother and the Daughter on the balcony, (left). Photo: © Denis de Marney/V&A Images, Victoria and Albert Museum, London.

Only the Lover remains, and luckily strikes it rich by finding a gold mine pointed out to him in a dream by his unfaithful fiancée. It's a huge joke that this digging sequence is on top of a stage trap that slowly lets him down as he digs deeper. Meanwhile, the Black King of this region, with his chamberlains and Witch Doctor have arrived in the same Kensington square to set up an embassy in the house vacated by the Rich Old Neighbour. Mother and Daughter are happy to be wooed by the African king but his designs upon the young woman are purely culinary. When the Lover turns up again, rich from his African gold mine, he discovers only a very large tureen with all that is left of her – the diamond ring she got from him and the diamond necklace from the Rich Old Neighbour.

The ballet tells its story very efficiently, with no need for a written synopsis. It's a thoroughly enjoyable piece of theatre. Monica Collingwood cuts out a picture of first-night dignitaries in the Crush Bar for her scrapbook and records her own presence 'in the shadows'.[47] Although Cyril Beaumont thinks the jokes are likely to wear thin, Lionel Bradley reports he still finds it enjoyable at his tenth viewing![48] Which set of inhabitants comes off worse in this satire, those of South Kensington or of the African jungle? Of course we are entitled to ridicule South Kensington for all its pretentions since Kensington can take care of itself, but is mocking Africa in a different category? Our Black King (Alexander Grant, blacked up) wears a quasi-military uniform and has some pretentions to adopting the niceties of European diplomacy.[49] His chamberlains are dressed in formal frock coats but wear African masks. We are encouraged to think that,underneath the external trappings, these are really unreconstructed savages who apparently cannot be 'civilised'. Perhaps in the private thoughts of some of our spectators, considering the viciousness of the Mau Mau insurgency in Kenya, this is not too far from the truth. Certainly it is noticeable that the plot, with its cannibal consumption of a young woman has some resemblance to Evelyn Waugh's novel, Black Mischief of 1932[50] so it is not too exceptional to enjoy this crude but amusing caricature of Africa.[51]

Is there any contradiction in simultaneously admiring the serious artistry of 'coloured' dancers from America, who are really very welcome and attractive visitors? Perhaps we become a little confused at what they show us. Back in November, Pearl Primus was here, putting on stage some of the dances she had learnt during her study trips to Africa.[52] If we want somehow to get an insight, from afar, into an authentic Africa (noble savages perhaps?) we are frustrated by the synthetic environment of the theatre, just a handful of dancers when we wanted to see whole tribes pounding out a rhythm.[53] Her own expressive dances get closer to what we expect from theatrical presentation. When she dances the poem where 'Strange Fruit' are lynched men hanging from trees in the southern States, we can recognise the artistry and be moved,[54] although there may be an underlying discomfort. Does this have anything to do with us? Certainly there are parts of London where pressures around housing and jobs could be tanking up resentment against large numbers of Caribbean and colonial African immigrants. One such place is north of the well-heeled Kensington Squares, but still in the borough, a slummy area called either North Kensington or Notting Hill. London has this Janus-headed quality of housing the splendid and the squalid within walking distance. It's just as well that that we don't expect anybody from there to attend the Opera House for Bonne-Bouche. A rumour of cannibalism could set the city alight![55]

Katherine Dunham and Company have recently been here from January to March at the Cambridge Theatre, another season in Peter Daubeny's continuing series of dance companies from around the world. Dunham certainly knows how to put on a show with a full company of singers, dancers and musicians and she can keep her audience coming for months. In this year's show, she moves around the Americas – a whole Brazilian Suite; tangos from Buenos Aires; her famous Shango from Trinidad and L'Ag'ya from Martinique; and finally she shows us black people dancing and singing in the USA, from plantation days to the 1920s 'Barrelhouse'.

She is adept at the theatricality of staged dances set on a framework of minimal story telling. Her theatrical intelligence makes her performances unique amongst the 'exotics' that London dance audiences love.[56] If there is any deeper message it is carefully wrapped up in pure enjoyment of 'the best revue in the world'.[57] It appears that John Cranko has tried to copy some of her dance movements for his African dances in *Bonne-Bouche*, but not very effectively.[58]

It so happens that British Caribbean people have their own dance company, Ballets Nègres, established in London in 1946, by the Jamaican dancer Berto Pasuka. This was some years before Dunham was seen in Britain. He wants to present 'Negro ballet', based upon African dance and music, as a serious art form. They spend much of their time touring in Europe but have a London season in September, not in the West End, but at the Twentieth Century Theatre in Westbourne Grove, north of the wealthy Kensington Osbert Lancaster imagines for *Bonne-Bouche* and east of the North Kensington slums where new West Indian immigrants are currently squeezing into rack-rented lodging houses. Pasuka spent several years studying Russian ballet in London, but some others of his dancers had little experience before joining. Some have come directly from the West Indies, but others are from long established black British families.

Pasuka puts on dance dramas with mainly Caribbean or African themes although a new work for this season, *Cabaret - 1920*, is set in Harlem. *Nine Nights*, another new work, is an example of his West Indian themes, in which the spirit of a dead child is put to rest by nine nights of ritual mixing African and Christian beliefs. Ballets Nègres has had a consistently good and appreciative press, although there are signs now that the standards of performance may be slipping in the face of a hectic schedule necessitated by lack of funds.[59] Should Ballets Nègres' message have particular meaning in Britain now in this current climate when there needs to be some understanding of how black and white citizens should get along with each other? Some of the dance dramas show how mixing is not easy. In *Blood*, the mixed-race wife of a white man is overcome by her racial heritage when experiencing a voodoo ceremony, and they both then become victims of the cult. In *They Came*, the figures of The Missionary, The Nurse, The Soldier and The Business Man clash with African culture but the outcome is a war which benefits no one. Some of us may view these dances in the understanding of their relevance to today in London. Pasuka may sometimes be accused non-specifically of 'propaganda'.[60] But for the most part, it is easier for us spectators to enjoy the dancing – uninhibited, exhibitionist and improvisational – assuming that this is, after all, the natural heritage of 'coloured' performers.[61]

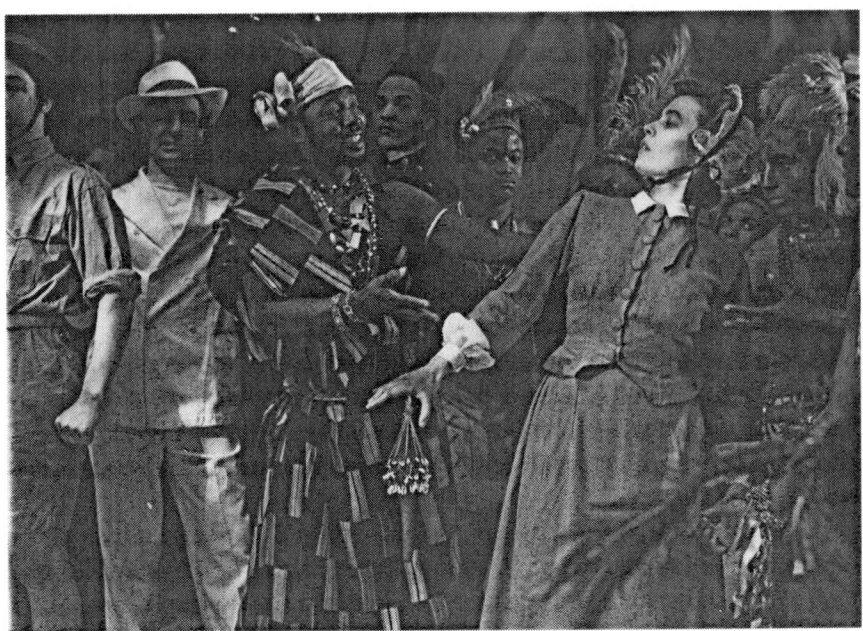

Ballets Nègres in *They Came* (chor. Pasuka, 1946), with Fernau Hall as The Business Man, Nat Laryea as The Chief and Patricia Clover as The Nurse. Photo: Angus McBean. MS Thr 581 411-13, Harvard Theatre Collection, Harvard University.

October
3rd : First UK atom bomb detonated off Australia.
6th : Tea rationing ends.
16th: Iran severs relations with UK over oil crisis.

November
1st: Testing of USA's first hydrogen bomb.

December
1st : 'Nutty Slack' (small coal) is taken off ration.
5th – 9th : Severe smog in London with possible deaths of 4,000 or more, penetrates Sadler's Wells Theatre and Royal Festival Hall.

On Sundays, ballet audiences are drawn to another real part of Kensington. In Ladbroke Road, near where it joins Kensington Park Road, is the Mercury Theatre, based in an old church hall. It has a tiny stage, made even more restricted by a staircase at the back, a permanent structure joining the stage to the studio behind and which has to be incorporated into every décor. Ballet Workshop started here last year as a platform for new choreography.[62] This is an off-shoot of Ballet Rambert, which has to spend most of its time (subsidised by the Arts Council) on provincial tours, rarely getting closer into the capital than the Lyric Theatre at Hammersmith. The Mercury can claim to be one of the earliest cradles of a British dance establishment, where the redoubtable Marie Rambert began her Ballet Club in 1931. Like Ballet Club, Ballet Workshop performs on Sundays to a membership audience, keeps production costs to a shoestring budget, and dancers only get a fraction of their expenses. But these are genuine productions, miniature works with a designer for décor and costumes, live music and very often a newly composed score. Ballet Workshop is therefore taken very seriously, with reviews in national papers as well as the dance press. Dancers also take it seriously. Somebody spends the intervals writing down the names of recognised members of the audience on the front of a programme.[63] These range through the Rambert family members, the principal and minor newspaper and journal critics, dancers who often perform with Ballet Workshop, dancers from Ballet Rambert and dancers from other companies. This is like a family reunion of dance insiders (critics, choreographers and dancers) and those of us who are just spectators can bask in their presence.

Rambert nurtured the first generation of British choreographers at the Ballet Club, including Frederick Ashton, Antony Tudor and Andrée Howard. Ballet Workshop attempts to do that for a new generation twenty years later and in keeping with the generational theme its directors are Rambert's daughter and son-in-law, Angela and David Ellis. The journalist Phyllis Manchester introduces the reasoning behind the Workshop in a programme note. This is about moving ballet on. 'An art can only live while it progresses.'

> Ballet Workshop does not promise a masterpiece every time. It does not say that there will not occasionally be a failure. ... If in five years' time Ballet Workshop has discovered one choreographer to take an established place in what is, perhaps, the rarest profession in the world; if it has produced three or four ballets worthy to be ranked with the very few that last a decade or more, then it may be said to have achieved what it now sets out with such hopes to do.

Take for example the performance witnessed by Lionel Bradley on 9 November 1952. It opens with a very slight work, about a road sweeper, *Le Balayeur*, rather pretentiously titled in French, with some business with a guardian angel and rescuing a drowning girl. This is not choreographically successful.[64]

Ouverture, with choreography by Jack Carter, is based on Marcel Proust's *Du Coté de chez Swann*. This would seem to be an impossible scenario, but it is saved by its intense atmosphere of haunting memories. The stage is divided in three, each with a Venetian blind in front of it so that illuminating the sections from within literally brings the memories into the light. (This appears to be a year for Venetian blinds!) The identity of the characters is deliberately kept vague. The Man lifts up a lamp in one part of the stage and at the same moment a woman we suppose to be His Mother lifts a lamp and starts to mount the stairs (the famous ones that obstruct the Mercury's stage put to ingenious use). We see episodes that move between pools of light, behind and in front of the louvered blinds. The Man sees Himself as a Child, greeting His Mother's guests. There is a central Woman in his life and also A Casual Encounter. An orchid brings lust and sex to mind. The interventions of The Friends seem difficult to fathom, unexplained and slightly sinister.[65]

The final dance in the programme is *Peepshow* by Walter Gore. He is certainly not a novice choreographer, with a history as a dancer with Rambert's Ballet Club and de Valois' Vic-Wells Ballet in the 1930s, and already quite a back-catalogue of works performed by a number of companies including Ballet Rambert. Since returning from working in Australia, he has been a strong supporter of Ballet Workshop, perhaps to help re-establish himself in London. Like *Ouverture, Peepshow* can only happen because of its ingenious stage set. The three dancers are seemingly pinned in their own place, each standing in a hole cut in a horizontal canvas but all we see at first are their legs performing balletic movements jerkily. There is a canvas across the stage obscuring their upper bodies. Now it moves down to show their upper bodies and hide the lower ones; they appear to be swimming. The obscuring of top or bottom of their bodies continues with some variations. At one point they all duck down and swim 'underwater' and at another one of them disappears to reappear in a different position. Finally the canvas is dropped and we get the full view of the dancers. The piece is really good fun, witty and fresh.[66]

This Ballet Workshop programme has done what it was intended for: at least one newish choreographer (Jack Carter) has been able to consolidate his craft with an adventurous approach.[67] It has already been a springboard for the career of Michael Charnley. This is something worth coming to Kensington for!

From the Windmill Theatre to the National Gallery

It's a short distance by foot from Great Windmill Street to Trafalgar Square but quite a cultural stretch from the Windmill Theatre to the National Gallery. The Windmill is the land of 'Revudeville', where the redoubtable owner, Mrs Laura Henderson, and her manager Vivian Van Damm instituted the novel idea of non-stop variety back in 1932, an all-day and evening show that can still be dipped into at will, 'come and go as you please'. Now the Windmill basks in its glorious wartime history as a theatrical enterprise declaring that in the Blitz, 'We Never Closed' (apart from the days of the 'phoney war' in September 1939 when there was a government decree against entertainments). Not only this, but the plucky little Windmill deserves a lot of praise since it manages to keep itself aloof from any of

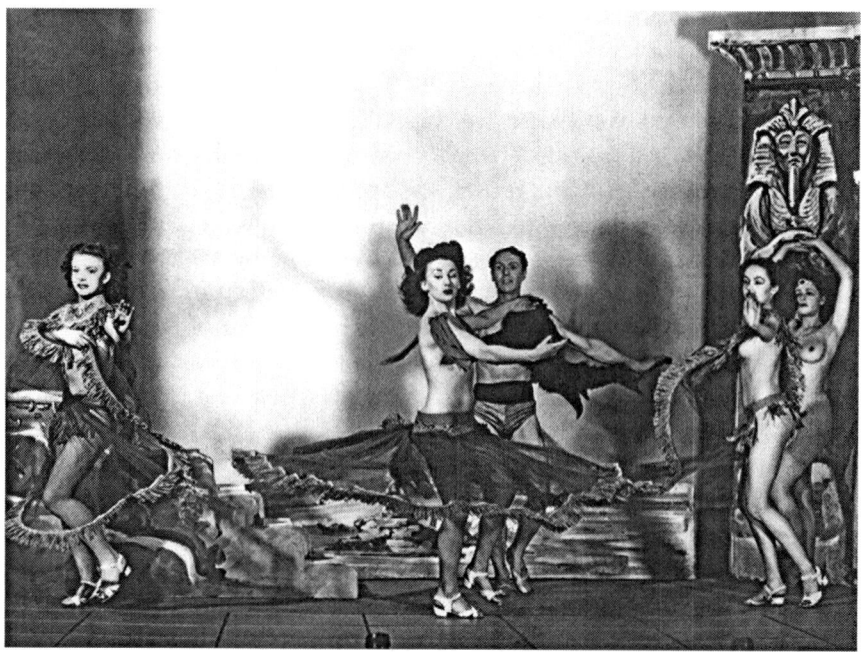

Joan Rock and Keith Lester (centre) perform in the number *Thou Shalt Not* at the Windmill Theatre, March 1947. Photo: © Central Press/Hulton Archive/Getty Images.

the nasty aspersions cast against it. It's a variety theatre, and its variety certainly is various, from comics and singing acts to ballets and the famous nude tableaux and fan dancers.[68] This is very much a male audience, here for the supposed salaciousness of the entertainment, but the Windmill takes its artistry seriously, forming a tight-knit community, or family, of impeccably behaved professionals: 'girls' downstairs, 'boys' upstairs and no visiting! Doris Barry, one of Markova's sisters, was a dancer here and was instrumental in persuading Henderson to financially support the Markova-Dolin Ballet in the 1930s. For artists, the Windmill is a very desirable venue, the chorus – two alternating companies, 'A Company' and 'B Company' – are paid full-time, including holidays and rehearsals. It appears that this land is a benevolent dictatorship.[69]

Keith Lester is ballet choreographer and principal dancer here, bringing his considerable experience of working with iconic dance figures of the twentieth century to what some might consider a rather debased form of entertainment. His past included training with Serafina Astafieva and Nicolas Legat; partnering Russian émigré ballerinas Lydia Kyasht, Tamara Karsavina and Olga Spessivtseva; performing in the company of Ida Rubinstein in Paris and in the Markova-Dolin Ballet in the 1930s (where he created his own version of *Pas de Quatre*); and forming the Arts Theatre Ballet in London in 1940 (which later merged with Ballet Rambert). At the

Windmill, Lester choreographs ballet scenes which sometimes use classical technique, and it would appear that he has been working to improve the technical ability of the dancers. He also choreographs dances (clothed) that happen around the ladies posing nude and in absolute stillness, the only way allowed by law. The fan dancers are also part of his province, with only two huge, tantalising ostrich feather fans to keep them decent, plus a couple of attendants called 'covers' who spoil the audience view of her body when she takes both fans away. Fantasy and mythical scenes give plenty of opportunity for showing off the chorus girls in fantastic costumes or part undressed: *Les Papillons*, *The Language of Flowers*, *Homage to Venus*, *Sea Idyll*.[70] Revudeville is the *risqué* version of what is happening at the Empire (where cine-variety is coming to a close this year) and another way of looking at the job of a dancer and of the characteristics of spectators. The fans queue politely here as elsewhere in London, but once the doors open there's the 'Windmill Steeplechase', vaulting over seats to get the coveted front rows. The really dedicated connoisseur can stay and see the whole show again... and again. This feels like a hundred miles from the stalls of the Royal Opera House, but is really one end of a continuum of dance performance in London.

That short walk to Trafalgar Square, skirting the theatreland of Shaftesbury Avenue and the Haymarket brings us to a place which is far removed from the back street entertainments of Great Windmill Street. Now we are close to the centre of London as capital city. Here is the great national hero on Nelson's Column, surrounded by the emblematic lions; the National Gallery (art heritage) and The National Portrait Gallery (with more national heroes and heroines). In November 1952 the final one of four mosaic pavements in the entrance lobbies of the National Gallery is unveiled. This project by the Russian artist Boris Anrep was started as long ago as 1928. A complicated character, Anrep was a lover of Russian poet Anna Akhmatova, and in London after 1917 was close to artistic circles including the Bloomsbury Group.

Steps lead up from the entrance to the half-landing where (considering that it is being trampled by visitors who never look down or understand what they walk on) it may be possible to see *The Awakening of the Muses*. Anrep's forte is to interpret classical themes from the viewpoint of his own time, and particularly from his own milieu amongst celebrities and artistic folk including the Bloomsbury set. So the Hollywood 'great' Greta Garbo, who wished to be 'left alone', is Melpomene, Muse of Tragedy. Lydia Lopokova, dancer with Diaghilev and later wife of economist and Bloomsburyite Maynard Keynes is Terpsichore, Muse of Dancing.

On landings at either side Anrep represents *The Labours of Life* and *The Pleasures of Life*. They show how much he, even as an émigré, has understood about the country. Pleasures are cricket, football, hunting, playing in the sea and Christmas pudding. Amongst the Labours is a panel of one of our Covent Garden porters representing Commerce, with a pile of baskets, soon to be balanced on his head in the time-honoured fashion.

In 1952, the final piece on the topmost landing is revealed, *The Modern Virtues*, twelve panels that say something about his view of Britain as well as making some highly personal statements. Anna Akhmatova is depicted as Compassion and he includes a representation of his own gravestone. Now it is more than twenty years since the beginning of the scheme and Anrep's choice of models for his virtues reflect the moment. Keenly topical is the current Prime Minister Winston Churchill, representing 'Defiance', in his wartime tin hat and dungarees, showing his V for Victory sign to a threatening monster before the White Cliffs of Dover. The philosopher Bertrand Russell is 'Lucidity'. The astronomer Fred Hoyle climbs towards the stars as 'Pursuit'. American film actress Loretta Young represents 'Compromise' as Anglo-American friendship. Edith Sitwell negotiates dangers as 'Sixth Sense' and T.S. Eliot, as 'Leisure', sits beside Loch Ness, with its monster making one of its very rare appearances.

Thinking back to the depictions of Britishness in last year's Festival of Britain, are there any similarities between that and this foreigner's view? Strangely, yes. In a way, the Lion and Unicorn pavilion is reflected here, in the fantasy figure ('Wonder') of Alice in Wonderland, being induced to new adventures by a mermaid ship's figurehead. In 'Humour', there is again a Britannia as in *Pineapple Poll*, (in this case the celebrity beauty Lady Diana Cooper), with her lion and Union Jack shield, crowning a figure of Punch from the satirical magazine. Again Britannia is allowed to be a comedienne.

But what we are really here to see is Margot Fonteyn. Sitting in the centre of the whole pavement she represents 'Delectation', calmly listening to Edward Sackville-West playing the harpsichord. Behind the harpsichord is a statue of Pomona, goddess of fruitful abundance[71] so in the iconography of this panel there is a suggestion that 'taste' and 'tastefulness' are profoundly sensory, even gustatory and Fonteyn is shown rapt and relishing the sensuousness of the music.

Perhaps there is also a small history lesson here. Frederick Ashton created a ballet on *Pomona*, danced by the Camargo Society. It was revived by the Vic-Wells Ballet in 1933 (although very rarely danced by Fonteyn) with new designs by Vanessa Bell, sister of Bloomsbury's Virginia Woolf. Edward Sackville-West was also a Bloomsbury insider. We can reflect here on the very close historical connections between ballet and London's intellectual life, and wonder if, in the 1950s, those connections have been broken. (Remember what Alan Dent says about ballet audiences!) But Fonteyn's position as a central cultural figure is confirmed amongst these representations of arts and sciences. She has already been hailed as one of the 'New Elizabethans' in *Picture Post*.[72] Flanked by 'Humour' and 'Wonder' on left and right, she seems to sit at the pivotal point of some of the modern virtues celebrated as typically British in the Lion and Unicorn pavilion of the South Bank Exhibition. Fans coming to view the mosaic may say she looks too detached, and too ethereal, colourless and rather stiff, which does not reflect the glowing warmth of her performance quality, which is set to illuminate 1953, Coronation year!

Notes

1　H.H. Princess Marie Louise (1956) *Memories of Six Reigns*, p.116.
2　Tyrone Guthrie, *News Chronicle*, 9 January 1952, p.2. Guthrie is right in insinuating the cultural popularity of musical theatre in the following decades. *The Boy Friend* (Sandy Wilson,1953) and *Salad Days* (Julian Slade and Dorothy Reynolds, 1954) were British productions in an arguably 'English' style which also had some transatlantic success. Arguably one would have to look much further forward to see the incorporation of 'light opera' into British musical theatre, for example in works by Tim Rice and Andrew Lloyd Webber in the 1970 and 80s. In *Cats* (1981) we see dance, music and words as equal partners.
3　Alan Dent, 'Haven't we had a little too much ballet?', *News Chronicle*, 29 January 1952.
4　Buckle wrote in *The Observer* on 20 January and 3 February. See Buckle's account of the controversy (1953) *The Adventures of a Ballet Critic*, pp.223-228. A letter exchange between Haskell and Dent is reprinted in *Ballet Annual*, 'Infamous Last Words on Ballet' (1953) *Ballet Annual, Seventh Issue*, pp.53 – 54.
5　See for example, Arnold Haskell, 'Infamous Last Words on Ballet' (1953) *Ballet Annual, Seventh Issue*, p.54.
6　On Guthrie see: Norman Lebrecht (2000) *Covent Garden: The Untold Story*, pp.44-46; on opera at Covent Garden , see Lebrecht, early chapters.
7　'Heads and Tails', *Picture Post*, 9 February 1952, p.22.
8　While the title of 'National Theatre' was settled on a company at the Old Vic in 1963, a dedicated theatre for the company was not opened until 1976. This building is sited on the south bank of the Thames, downstream of Waterloo Bridge and not included in the Southbank Centre although contiguous along the embankment from a walker's point of view.
9　Pendennis, 'Table Talk', *The Observer*, 13 January 1952, p.5.
10　The designs were by John Piper (*Harlequin in April*) and Isabel Lambert (*Tiresias*), both distinguished painters.
11　The roof and dome were destroyed by fire in 1956.
12　The market was taken over by a public body, the Covent Garden Authority in 1962 and was moved away to Battersea in 1973.

13 For the circumstances of the acquisition of the Royal Opera House, see: Norman Lebrecht (2000) *Covent Garden: The Untold Story*, pp.38-47.

14 For architectural and administrative histories of the Royal Opera House see: F.H.W. Sheppard, ed., *Survey of London: volume 35: The Theatre Royal, Drury Lane, and the Royal Opera House, Covent Garden* (1970), URL: http://www.british-history.ac.uk/source.aspx?pubid=1053. For Covent Garden Market see: F.H.W. Sheppard, ed., *Survey of London: volume 36: Covent Garden* (1970), URL: http://www.british-history.ac.uk/source.aspx?pubid=362.

15 Anatole Chujoy (1952) 'Four Opera Houses: London', *Ballet Annual, Sixth Issue*, pp.89-90.

16 Peter Williams, 'Editorial: How wide is the ocean?' *Dance and Dancers*, September 1952, p.5.

17 Caryl Brahms, 'I Blame Balanchine', *Ballet Today*, August 1952, pp.4-5.

18 Edwin Denby, 'New York City's Ballet', *Ballet*, August 1952, p.33.

19 'Commentary', *Ballet*, September 1952, p.5.

20 See Cyril Beaumont 'New York City Ballets Part III: Two of Robbins', *Ballet*, August 1952, pp.10-12.

21 Caryl Brahms, 'I Blame Balanchine', *Ballet Today*, August 1952, p.4.

22 'Nothing Barred in this Cage', *Picture Post*, 26 July 1952, pp.38-40.

23 *The Cage* is performed to Stravinsky's *Concerto in D for String Orchestra* (1946). Lionel Bradley, Ballet Bulletins, 7 July, and 13, 14 August 1952.

24 Lionel Bradley, Ballet Bulletins, 21 July 1952.

25 Peter Williams, 'Editorial: How wide is the ocean?', *Dance and Dancers*, September 1952, p.5.

26 Clive Barnes insisted *Cakewalk* was popular with audiences: 'Swing high – sink low', *Dance and Dancers*, September 1952, pp.12-15; but Buckle thought it was only the anti-Balanchine press that valued these Americana pieces, whereas seasoned ballet-goers recognised they were trifles ('Commentary', *Ballet*, September 1952, p.5).

27 Clive Barnes overheard this. 'Swing high – sink low', *Dance and Dancers*, September 1952, p.14.

28 *Theme with Four Variations [According to the Four Temperaments] for string orchestra and piano* (1940).

29 My analysis of *Four Temperaments* is based on the 1977 performance by the New York City Ballet in the Dance in America series, available on DVD, *Choreography by Balanchine*.

30 Edwin Denby, 'New York City's Ballet', *Ballet*, August 1952, p.34.

31 *Picture Post*, 28 June 1952, pp.4-5.

32 'Scenery Projection for Festival Ballet', *Ballet Today*, August 1952, p.16; Julian Braunsweg (1973) *Ballet Scandals*, pp.135-137. The London County Council, owning the Royal Festival Hall, encouraged Festival Ballet to become a regular attraction, with preferential rates.

33 Pamela Fletcher, 'Festival Ballet is a Real Tonic', *Ballet Today*, September 1952, p.6.

34 'Festival Ballet at the Royal Festival Hall', *Ballet Annual, Eighth Issue*, p.7.

35 Anton Dolin, 'Psychological Ballets', *The Dancing Times*, October 1952, p.21.

36 At the first performance, Lionel Bradley describes a loose net curtain here, but subsequent photographs show the effect of blinds.

37 'Rolled up jeans are 'jazz style'', *Picture Post*, 23 June 1951, p.23. The designs of *Symphony for Fun* were by Tom Lingwood, who had already made designs for Ballet Workshop.

38 The music made reference to a number of American musical genres. Gillis is regarded

as a composer with a nationalist output, whose work included other nostalgic 'Americana' themes. Charnley took the symphony's four movements in reverse order, but it was not sufficiently well-known for this to have been noticed by critics.

39 This analysis of *Symphony for Fun* was based upon the following primary sources: Peter Williams, 'Symphony for Fun', *Dance and Dancers*, October 1952, p.13; Pamela Fletcher, 'Symbolising Youth of 1952', *Ballet Today*, October 1952, p.6; John Hall, 'First Performance of Michael Charnley's *Symphony for Fun*', *Ballet*, October 1952, pp.28-29; Lionel Bradley, Ballet Bulletins, 1 September 1952; Personal communication from Peter Bassett, 10 January 1999; Ann Barzel film collection, approx. 3 mins. black and white, silent film, filmed Chicago 1954, Jerome Robbins Dance Division, NYPL, *MGZIC 9-3598.

40 'They lost their hair, *Dance and Dancers*, October 1952, p.17.

41 Pamela Fletcher, 'Symbolising Youth of 1952', *Ballet Today*, October 1952, p.6.

42 'The Sitter Out', *The Dancing Times*, October 1952, p.7.

43 The Telecinema survived the destruction of the South Bank Exhibition and reopened in October 1952 as the first National Film Theatre. The stereoscopic films produced for the Festival of Britain – *Now is the Time, Around is Around, A Solid Explanation, The Distant Thames* – were shown there. It is not clear whether *The Black Swan* was also shown at the Telecinema.

44 Peter Brinson wrote the film scenario. A viewing copy is held at the National Film Archive but without the 3D effect. 'The Black Swan', *Dance and Dancers*, June 1952, p.13; John Hall, 'Two Ballet Films', *Ballet*, July 1952, pp.16-19 ; Peter Brinson 'Filming Ballet in three dimensions', *Dance and Dancers*, August 1952, pp.18-19.

45 For example, *Façades and Faces* (1950), London: John Murray

46 Alexander Bland, 'Ballet: Tit-Bit', *The Observer*, 6 April 1952, p.6.

47 '*Bonne-Bouche*', *Tatler and Bystander*, 23 April 1952, pp.198-199.

48 Cyril Beaumont, 'Bonne Bouche', *Ballet*, June 1952, pp.33-43; Lionel Bradley, Ballet Bulletins, 18 September 1952.

49 'Blacking up' had previously occurred on the ballet stage, notably in Frederick Ashton's and Buddy Bradley's *High Yellow* at the Camargo Society in 1932; and Andrée Howard's *The Sailor's Return* for Ballet Rambert in 1947. In the latter, Sally Gilmour portrayed the tragic outcome for an African princess brought home to England as the wife of a sailor.

50 This is noticed in: JHM, '"Bonne Bouche": New Ballet at Covent Garden', *The Manchester Guardian*, 5 April 1952, p.3; 'Sadler's Wells Ballet: "Bonne-Bouche"', *The Times*, 5 April 1952, p.3. Cannibalism can now be recognised as a trope, used frequently and sometimes unconsciously in western literature but ultimately justifying colonialism and racism. It contrasts this taboo in 'civilised' nations with the supposed breaking of this human taboo in 'primitive' societies, therefore questioning shared humanity. Another example is quoted in the autobiographical novel by V S Naipaul, *The Enigma of Arrival* (1987) in which all that is left of the young woman is 'a twenties costume draped on a wooden cross, like a scarecrow' (p.253).Culturally embedded cannibalism, for example in New Guinea, has been for ritual purposes rather than to satisfy hunger.

51 Cranko was a South African but I do not imply that his views were any more racist than the casual and unrecognised racism prevalent through the cannibalism myths on which this ballet was based. In 1960 he was a signatory to a statement by 'distinguished South Africans' deploring the policy of apartheid. See: 'London Letter: South African isolation', *The Guardian*, 31 May 1960, p.8.

52 Primus was invited to perform at the Royal Command Performance on 29 October

1951 before commencing her season: Arthur Todd, 'Meet Pearl Primus', *Ballet Today*, November 1951, pp.11-12.

53 J.M.M. 'Negro Dancers', *The Manchester Guardian*, 2 November 1951, p.5.

54 Arnold Haskell (1953) 'Outstanding Events of the Year: Pearl Primus', *Ballet Annual, Seventh Issue*, p.11.

55 On 30 August 1958, in the midst of a heat wave, the Notting Hill Race Riots broke out in this area. There were local tensions between black and white residents, exacerbated by neo-nazi Mosleyite factions and gangs of Teddy boys. Attacks on black people and properties continued for a week. It was fortunate that no one was killed during these events. There is evidence that news of murders committed by the Mau Mau in Kenya was already heightening tensions in the early 1950s (Robert Winder (2004) *Bloody Foreigners: The Story of Immigration to Britain*, p.365).

56 Arnold Haskell (1953) 'Outstanding Events of the Year: Katherine Dunham', *Ballet Annual, Seventh Issue*, pp.18-19.

57 Richard Buckle, 'Dunham's Return', *The Observer*, 13 January 1952, p.6.

58 Clive Barnes, 'Bonne-Bouche', *Dance and Dancers*, May 1952, p.14.

59 Peter Brinson, 'Ballets Nègres at the Twentieth Century Theatre', *Ballet*, October 1952, pp.30-31. Ballets Nègres ceased to function in 1953.

60 'Twentieth Century: Ballets Nègres', *The Stage*, 11 September 1952.

61 This reductionist view can be detected in the following review: A.E., 'Ballets Nègres at the Twentieth Century Theatre', *The New Statesman*, 20 September 1952. For a supportive assessment in the early years of the company see: Audrey Williamson (1948) 'Negro Ballet', *Ballet Renaissance*, pp.83-87.

62 Ballet Workshop ceased operations in 1955 after the Arts Council refused to give financial support.

63 Programmes available in Rambert Dance Company Archive.

64 'The Sitter Out', *The Dancing Times*, December 1952, p.132; Clive Barnes, 'Ballet Workshop: Le Balayeur', *Dance and Dancers*, January 1953, p.24.

65 'The Sitter Out', *The Dancing Times*, November 1952, pp.131-132; Clive Barnes, 'New Ballets: Ouverture', *Dance and Dancers*, January 1953, pp.12-13; Frank Jackson (1953) *They Make Tomorrow's Ballet*, pp.5-6.

66 'The Sitter Out', *The Dancing Times*, November 1952, p.69; Clive Barnes, 'New Ballet: Peepshow', *Dance and Dancers*, December 1952, p.17.

67 Jack Carter previously had four compositions in Ballet Workshop. *Ouverture* went into the repertoire of Ballet Rambert as *Past Recalled*.

68 Mrs Henderson died in 1944 but Van Damm and subsequently his daughter continued Revudeville until 1964. A number of comedy turns who appeared at the Windmill became household names in Britain: for example, Jimmy Edwards, Bruce Forsythe, Harry Secombe, Peter Sellers, Arthur English.

69 Keith Lester, 'Dancers at the Windmill', *The Dancing Times*, November 1964, p.91; Peter Williams 'Ballet in the Kingdom of Revudeville', *Dance and Dancers*, April 1952, p.17.

70 'The Windmill', *The Stage*, 17 July and 13 November 1952, p.5.

71 Lois Oliver (2004) *Boris Anrep: The National Gallery Mosaics*, London: National Gallery Company, inside back cover.

72 'Picture Post Picks the New Elizabethans', *Picture Post*, 19 April 1952, pp.36-43.

CHAPTER FOUR

1953: A CROWNING GLORY

February
3rd : East coast storms and high tide kill 300.
5th : Sweet rationing ends.

March
5th : In USSR the death of Stalin is announced.
18th : Fonteyn returns to Covent Garden after 5 months' absence due to diphtheria.
24th : Death of Queen Mary.

Queen Sees Ideal Homes 1953, British Pathé Newsreel,
5 March 1953

A perfect scale model of the Coronation State Coach complete with full retinue is the high spot of the 1953 Daily Mail Ideal Homes Exhibition in London. When Her Majesty the Queen and the Duke of Edinburgh visit the show they pay special attention to the magnificent cavalcade which is more than a hundred feet in length. The ideal garden for the ideal home is another attraction at the Exhibition. Lakes, lawns, fountains and hundreds of beautiful flowers have all been arranged by gardening experts. Officials accompany the Queen and the Duke in their tour of the gardens which are lit by artificial sunlight. Some homes you can order straight from the stands. [Sign reads: Ministry of Housing and Local Government: The People's House, 1953. Way in.] It's the first time for fourteen years this has been possible, so salesmen are standing by for a big rush. Her Majesty inspects one of them. Labour and space-saving devices equip all the new houses, many of which can be ready for occupation before winter. British craftsmen combine ingenuity and grace in this year's ideal home.[1]

A walk around Olympia and backhome for television

In the National Hall of Olympia, a village of full sized houses in modern design is on show; some will be erected by local authorities and some can be bought for £2,200 for erection elsewhere, and now, for the first time postwar it will be possible to get a building licence without a lot of red tape. If the postwar housing crisis is still not over, at least we are being encouraged to imagine it away! As we walk through the exhibits, few of us can expect to possess these fresh and functional spaces, all designed externally and internally for specific family needs (e.g. 'a husband and wife with one child, a little girl of four').[2] Most of us will dream of the labour-saving future they hold out to us and of beautifully coordinated furnishings[3] – then go to buy jam and pastries from the 'village market' run by the Women's Institute, or buy sweets and chocolates (now off-ration!) at one of the other 'village shops'. As we hunt through the other floors for something useful to take away (perhaps the ultimately squeezable mop) we may begin to wonder where the televisions are, since they do not appear to be in the furnishings of the ideal homes. This must be the year of the television! New sets with bigger seventeen inch screens are on the market. Nearly the whole country has access to a transmitter therefore one would assume that no new home at Olympia would be complete without a television, but this appears not to be so. Perhaps the designers are confused by the apparent lack of function in the television set. Or perhaps it's because televisions sets are so ugly, in massive dark wood boxes, not at all in the light, graceful style our contemporary designers favour.

*   *   *   *   *

It's Good Friday, 3 April, and this is the third performance of *Les Sylphides* broadcast on television in the last few years. Back in 1946, when television resumed after the war, it was pretty much a London affair but since then the national coverage has been growing fast, extending north and west. Television producers have found that dance is a rich store of entertainment, but it hasn't been easy for television to adapt technically. The space of the television studio and the space of the television screen are tiny in comparison to the normal dance spaces. This is not like film. The huge expanse of the film sound-stage (remember *Tales of Hoffmann?*) is not available in the BBC's London Lime

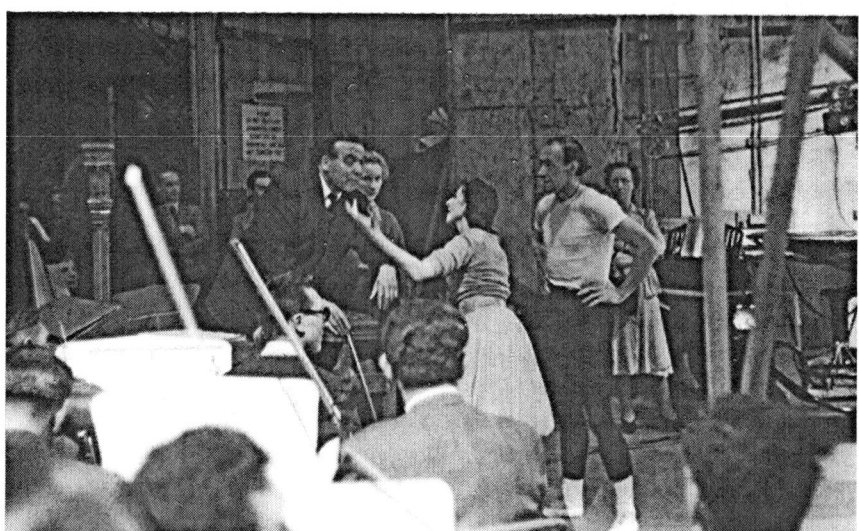

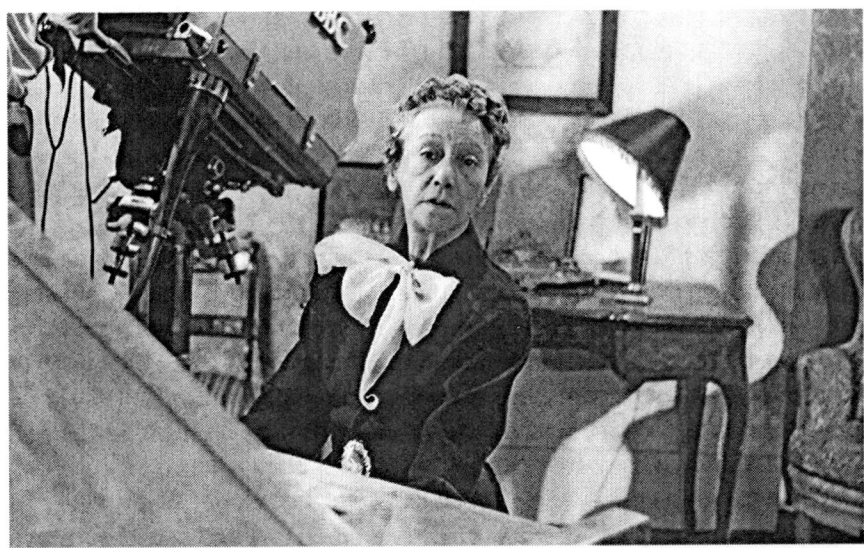

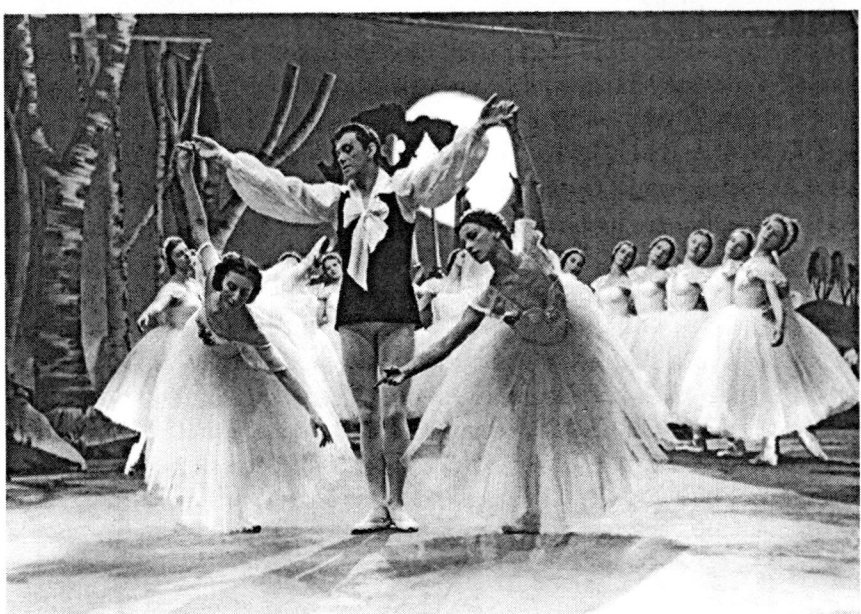

Studio images of the BBC television broadcast of *Les Sylphides*, 3 April 1953. Alicia Markova in animated discussion with conductor Eric Robinson while John Field looks on. Tamara Karsavina faces the tv camera. John Field supports Alicia Markova and Violetta Elvin in the television studio set. Photos: G.B.L. Wilson. © Royal Academy of Dance/ ArenaPAL.

Grove Studio. The programmes go out live which compounds all the technical difficulties of keeping dancers in shot. There are complaints about losing feet and heads, which makes nonsense of a dance production! Usually there is a live orchestra but space constraints force it to be in another studio. And yet, could this be a new beginning for this art form, brought into the domestic arena on BBC Television, the single channel of the national broadcaster? Since 1950 there have been television versions of *Giselle*, *Sleeping Beauty* and *Swan Lake*, plus two programmes of short works from Ballet Rambert, one from the British Dance Theatre and numerous short programmes of ballet or national dance, six of these just in the last twelve months.[4] In addition *Ballet for Beginners* has run four series of regular programmes since 1949, soon to be a fifth series, telling the general public about ballet and what to look for in performance. If dance on the little screen and dance on the big stage can combine, this could be a way of really expanding the audience.

This performance of *Les Sylphides* is certainly the best one we have seen. It manages to achieve a consistent tone of romantic reverie throughout, even when giving historical information. This blend is only achieved through a rather inspired idea that the beloved Russian ballerina, Tamara Karsavina, should do the introduction as if remembering with the help of a programme and her scrapbook, that first Paris performance in 1909 when she danced it with Pavlova and Nijinsky in Diaghilev's first season. This simple device shows up the ghastliness of the stilted voice-overs we have had in previous television ballet productions. She appears to be in her own drawing room (a studio set). As she reminisces, the French windows open to reveal a fantasy garden, a dreamy landscape of memory. There is a clearing in a birch wood, and a romantic ecclesiastical ruin in the background is bathed in the light of a full moon. Karsavina intones the names of the dancers as if they would be her dream cast for a 1953 production – John Field as the Poet, with Svetlana Beriosova, Violetta Elvin and Alicia Markova, the first three currently from the Sadler's Wells Ballet, which makes for some consistency of approach. Markova, of course is still considered the epitome of the balletic-romantic style, as in her interpretations of *Giselle* and of Taglioni in *Pas de Quatre*.

The studio space is tight but somehow they have managed to fit in the full *corps de ballet* of sixteen. Frustratingly, the beauty of their groupings disappears into a sea of tulle except when a raised camera angle temporarily relieves the crush and shows a little more of the patterning. The principal dancers make us forget their restrictions. There is plenty of atmosphere heightened by close-ups of rapt faces. Beriosova is deeply absorbed within the rhythm of the Valse. In the Prelude, Markova dreamily hovers, listening to the sounds of the night. Field's Poet seems immersed in a supernatural dream from which he may never escape. Despite restrictions, Elvin appears to soar across the diagonals of the space in the Mazurka, and instead of making an exit as she would on stage she flits between the birch trees behind the *corps de ballet* to reach her next corner. This makes sense of the action and creates another image, and an unexpected one, for people who know the ballet. We are reminded that the performing space in not bounded by the edge of the stage but only by the edge of the imagination. The ballet ends as the camera draws back through the window, indoors to Karsavina and her memories.[5]

May
29th : Conquest of Everest by a Commonwealth expedition.

June
2nd : Coronation of Queen Elizabeth II at Westminster Abbey

Walking the Coronation Route

After leaving Westminster Abbey, the Procession takes a long route of about one and a half hours around Central London to achieve maximum public display, marching, driving and trotting in symbolic order. Four British military bands head the parade, followed by the 'Colonial Contingents', detachments of police, air force, army and navy representing overseas territories, colonies, and protectorates.[6] The global scope is stunning. To give just a few examples: there are parties from Europe (Cyprus, Malta, Gibraltar); the Caribbean (Bahamas, Barbados, Jamaica, Windward and Leeward Islands); Pacific islands (Fiji, Solomon Islands); Asia and South-East Asia (Hong Kong, Malaya, Singapore); Africa (Kenya, Somaliland, Rhodesia); and the Falkland Islands in the South Atlantic. These are followed by the massed forces of the Commonwealth countries – Ceylon, Pakistan, South Africa, New Zealand, Australia, Canada, but not of India as it is a republic – and then by representatives of all the British armed services. Now, as the carriage processions commence, each with its escorts and outriders, we get some idea of the careful arrangement of precedence. In the Carriage Procession of Colonial Rulers, four open carriages carry seven Sultans, and Queen Salote of Tonga who continues to beam and wave to the crowd despite the pouring rain. The Carriage Procession of Prime Ministers comes next, with a carriage for each Commonwealth prime minister culminating in the carriage of Prime Minister Winston Churchill of the United Kingdom. Then come the royalty: Princes and Princesses of the Blood Royal in three carriages and the Queen Mother and Princess Margaret in the Glass Coach. Finally there is the build-up to the Queen herself in the Gold Coach pulled by eight grey horses, the anticipation brought to a crescendo by the line upon line of named dignitaries, aides, royal staff, and leaders of the armed forces who precede her.

From the Abbey, the procession wends its way through streets and past stands, hung with red and gold pennants, banners and union flags. Up

Whitehall (a pompous enclave of departments of state) it goes. By way of Pall Mall, and St James's Street, it reaches Piccadilly, where it passes number 145, now bombed, where the Queen spent some of her childhood. At Hyde Park Corner it turns northwards into Hyde Park (in front of the stand where choreographer Frederick Ashton has been sitting in the rain since 7am)[7] up to Marble Arch. Turning east into Oxford Street and then south into Regent's Street the procession takes in the commercial centre of London with its great shops (Selfridges, Marshall and Snelgrove, John Lewis, Liberty's) every window crammed with faces and the front of Selfridges in particular is overloaded with decorations.

At Piccadilly Circus, it moves into London's theatreland. Right by the statue of Eros is the Criterion Theatre where a play called *The Young Elizabeth* appropriately tells the story of the first Queen Elizabeth in her youth. The theatre itself is underground; some of us remember this made it perfect for radio broadcasting during the war. In the Haymarket, the procession passes between two theatres facing each other. At the Theatre Royal they are currently playing *The Apple Cart* by George Bernard Shaw and opposite at Her Majesty's Theatre, the American musical *Paint Your Wagon*, choreography by Agnes de Mille, has been having great success despite its sordid story of sex-hungry miners in the gold rush.

A right wheel and the procession is swinging down The Mall. It's a straight road now, all the way to Buckingham Palace, passing other royal residences, Marlborough House where Queen Mary lived until her so-recent death, and Clarence House where the Queen, as Princess Elizabeth, set up home after her marriage. The Mall is crossed by four metal arches, surmounted by the Lion and Unicorn, with a coronet hanging beneath the apex of each. If 'the Lion and the Unicorn are fighting for the crown' as in the children's rhyme, no such thing is happening here. The symbolic order is perfect and so the Gold Coach passes beneath these triumphal arches to reach the Palace and the anticipated balcony appearance.

We watch it all in person if we are lucky, or else on television or at the cinema. There are even said to be fifty television sets in the Festival Pleasure Gardens at Battersea, now open for its third season.[8]

Many of us come back to walk the route, to enjoy the decorations and the spectacle in memory or imagination, thinking again about the meaning of it all. What about the connections between the royal family and establishing the art form of ballet in Britain? Does it ever seem to princesses and queens watching ballets on stage that the performance throws back to them images that echo their own lives? Do they see the female stars on stage as reflecting something similar to the position of royal women, and do they see the performance of ballet and the performance of royal duties as similarly constrained by hierarchies and conventions? If ballet is in some ways a little parallel kingdom to the massive one of the state, it also has its queen. There are many aspirants to the supreme position of *prima ballerina assoluta*, the ballerina of her generation that transcends all others, truly like its monarch. Here we have had Markova and now Fonteyn acceding to that throne. What makes the *assoluta*? It's more than technique. Part of it may be the 'inner radiance' similar to what flows from the new Queen. The *assoluta* must have 'an inherent nobility of mind and a natural aristocracy, both on and off the stage.'[9] Markova and Fonteyn are always conscious of that perfection of dress and deportment (fashion, furs, hats, make-up) which they must present to the public outside the stage door. Like royalty, they are always on show.

The attachment of our female royalty to ballet goes back a long way. As a teenage princess in the 1830s, Queen Victoria attended the principal London theatres for opera and ballet. Later, as Queen she was also a spectator, although her attendance was rather more formal. Despite the depredations of time, and conflagrations that have been as frequent as bushfires in theatre history, the theatrical footprints of those places in London still seem indestructible in 1953 – Drury Lane, Covent Garden, and Her Majesty's in the Haymarket which was passed by the Coronation Procession.

Queen Victoria experienced the height of the romantic ballet in London in the 1830s and 1840s. She wrote about theatre expeditions in her diary and sometimes sketched her favourite performers including Marie Taglioni in *La Bayadère* and Pauline Duvernay in *The Sleeping Beauty*.[10] Her governess, Baroness Lehzen, helped her to dress small dolls in the costumes of the ballets. The dolls were the subject of an article in *The Strand Magazine*, in September 1892, with footnotes which had apparently been contributed by the Queen herself as corrections to the text.[11] And of course Queen Victoria saw one of the first performances of Jules Perrot's *Pas de Quatre* in 1845 with four of the most celebrated ballerinas of the day: Marie Taglioni, Fanny Cerrito, Carlotta Grisi and Lucile Grahn.[12]

After retiring from the stage, Taglioni gave dancing and deportment lessons between 1872 and 1880 in premises in Connaught Square, London. The royal family's connection with Taglioni continued in the exclusive classes she gave for royal and noble children. An insight comes from Margaret Rolfe who described and sketched the classes.[13] Amongst her classmates was Princess May of Teck, a great-granddaughter of King George III, who would become Queen Mary, consort of King George V.[14]

Taglioni's classes were a rather strange mixture of callisthenic exercises, deportment, etiquette, fancy and social dancing. Pupils learned the deep and half curtsy, gradated according to rank; how to enter and leave the room when royalty was present; how to manage a train. Such were the skills they would eventually need when being presented at court. Dances with scarves, tambourines and fans were also part of Taglioni's curriculum, as well as some simple ballet movements like *ronds de jambes*. Princess May did not enjoy dance classes, which she also had to endure with the former dancer, now society dancing master, Louis d'Egville. The circuit of the room in curtsy practice, and the parade with a train made from one of Taglioni's heavy tablecloths were torture for her shy nature.[15] But to watch others embodying the noble classicism with such style on stage, and curtsying so gracefully to her, seems quite another matter.

In 1921, now Queen Mary with King George V, she attended a gala performance of Diaghilev's production of *The Sleeping Princess* at the Alhambra Theatre, Leicester Square. Did she see in this old ballet of Imperial Russia, with its courtly precedence and preoccupation with royal marriage, a connection with her own life? Possibly this ballet made more sense to her than to the bourgeois intellectuals from Bloomsbury who followed Diaghilev for his modernism and found this ballet from the court of Imperial Russia to be retrogressive. In 1928, she became patron of the Association of Teachers of Operatic Dancing, ballet teachers who wanted to raise the standard of technical training. The Association became truly 'royal' in 1936 with a charter as the Royal Academy of Dancing. Queen Mary remained loyal to the Academy and gave her splendid presence to galas, including one by Festival Ballet at the Stoll in 1950. Press photographs from such occasions make her appear very formal but it seems otherwise. There are stories of her chatting about her lessons with Taglioni, telling Markova and Dolin about her experience learning a mazurka, and even showing a few steps; or that, attending the theatre with a royal party, she danced a 'minuet' with her brother, the Earl of Athlone.[16] (Both Teck brothers attended Taglioni's classes where they were very naughty, according to Margaret Rolfe.[17])

Dedicated patronage of ballet in this country mainly comes from the female royals, but Anton Dolin remembers that the Duke of Connaught (Queen Victoria's son, Prince Arthur), was very interested in Diaghilev's company when it was based in Monte Carlo.[18] This may have been because of his musical interest: he was President of the Royal Academy of Music.

A royal person staunchly supporting ballet in 1953 is Princess Marie Louise, a granddaughter of Queen Victoria. Since she had an unhappy marriage to a minor German prince annulled in 1900, she has lived back in England, devoted to good and charitable causes. Her own childhood dance classes, held in the Albert Institute, Windsor, were not as public and traumatic as Queen Mary's.[19] She became the patron of the newly formed Festival Ballet in 1950 and apparently sends her used court gowns to be cut up for costume decorations.[20] Her interest in ballet goes back to the 1930s. Strange as it may seem, she was a friend of that Mrs Laura Henderson, proprietor of the Windmill Theatre of Revudeville fame who also financially backed the Markova-Dolin Ballet. They came together to Markova-Dolin Company performances.[21]

Taking the opportunity to write about royal patronage of ballet in 1953, Anton Dolin believes that, of all the royal ladies, Queen Elizabeth the Queen Mother has seen most ballet and Princess Margaret, President of the Sadler's Wells Foundation (the body owning Sadler's Wells Theatre), is most knowledgeable. Following the death of Queen Mary, the new Queen Elizabeth has consented to become patron of the Royal Academy of Dancing in her place. It's not just their names that royal ladies contribute. In the gloomy days of austerity, the royal women add glamour and reassuring affluence to ballet galas, even for most people who only see the occasions on newsreels or read about them in the newspapers. Glitter on their gowns, shining pure white mink capes, and diamonds – diamonds in tiaras, diamonds in necklaces, diamonds in bracelets, diamonds in earrings![22]

*   *   *   *   *

the isle is full of noises,
Sounds, and sweet airs, that give delight and hurt not.[23]

The reviewer from *The Times* reflects in these appropriately Shakespearean words on all the sounds and delights of Coronation Day, which concludes with a ballet gala at the Royal Opera House.[24] Much to the regret of ballet interests, this is not to be a royal gala.[25] It begins with Act II of *Lac des Cygnes* (as *Swan Lake* is currently called here). At 9.00 pm Queen Elizabeth's Coronation broadcast is played to the auditorium, just as it is heard on radios at home and overseas. Directly the response from the Sadler's Wells Ballet follows, *Homage to the Queen*, a new ballet by Frederick Ashton. The programme ends with Ashton's *Façade*, set to music William Walton composed to accompany Edith Sitwell's rhythmical verses of that name.

The dual themes of the gala are of honouring the past in the present and of honouring female sovereignty, which is very much at one with the day on the streets and in Westminster Abbey. Past and present together equal the promise of continuity. The ballet community sees itself reflected in this, not only because of its royal patronage. In *Dance and Dancers*, Peter Williams writes in four parts a history of ballet in Britain that parallels the life of Queen Elizabeth. The story he tells is of birth, childhood, youth, coming-of-age and dedication to the nation. The year of the Queen's birth (1926) was the year of Ashton's little ballet *A Tragedy of Fashion* in intimate revue at Hammersmith, a success that raised the possibility that his mentor Marie Rambert could form a company. It was also the year when Ninette de Valois opened her Academy of Choregraphic [sic] Art in London, leading eventually to the institutions as we see them in 1953: the Sadler's Wells

Ballet School and companies at Covent Garden and Sadler's Wells Theatre. By the age of ten the young Princess Elizabeth was heir presumptive to the throne after the abdication of her uncle Edward VIII; and Markova had departed the Sadler's Wells Ballet leaving Margot Fonteyn heir presumptive to the supreme ballerina position. In the war years ballet companies kept performing in London, even during air raids, and the royal family remained too. So the late 1940s brought popularity and maturity, Princess Elizabeth married and a mother, and another kind of marriage solemnised between Sadler's Wells Ballet and Covent Garden.[26] Tonight, on the Opera House stage, past and present are made explicit in the programming: the classical tradition of *Swan Lake* is represented by Fonteyn, our current balletic queen, and Robert Helpmann, the first male star of the company in the 1930s and 40s, still a wonderful dance-actor, but now being superseded by better ballet technicians. Ashton's premiere for this specific occasion is followed by *Façade*, one of his earliest and most enduring successes. A period piece from the 1930s, its gaiety is so 'tongue in cheek' and 'English'.

As the audience hears at Covent Garden and next to radios everywhere, the Queen speaks of 'the living strength and Majesty of the Commonwealth and Empire, of societies old and new, of lands and races different in history and origins but all, by God's will, united in spirit and in aim'. She speaks of 'our message to the world', those British virtues that spread outwards: the rule of law, tolerance and free speech. 'I have in sincerity pledged myself to your service, as so many of you are pledged to mine. Throughout all my life and with all my heart I will strive to be worthy of your trust.'[27]

The ballet programme on this night presents no less than seven balletic queens on stage. Margot Fonteyn is a peerless Swan Queen in *Lac des Cygnes*, at her Lakeside meeting with Siegfried. Then, in *Homage to the Queen*, queens of Earth, Water, Fire and Air, with their consorts and retinues appear, and in a majestic finale we meet representations of both Queen Elizabeth I and Queen Elizabeth II.

Homage to the Queen is a newly commissioned score by Malcolm Arnold (very appropriate to have an English composer) and also one that echoes the nineteenth-century form of *The Sleeping Beauty*'s last act with its processions, divertissements and homage finale. There is a processional entry for all the four queens and their courts. The queens are classically attired in tutus though the *corps de ballets* have longer skirts, wide at the hips, suggesting the shape of an Elizabethan gown. Colours are appropriate to the elements: rose, brown, blue, red and bluish white. The queens and their consorts wear crowns, of course. The setting is of bluish gauzes, receding into the background with a far view of trees studded with candles.

Earth has birdsong in the music, a sense of opening landscape and amusing jazziness in the score, with many little steps for its Queen, Nadia

Nerina, emphasising the ground. Water brings musical sounds of dripping, floods and waterfalls, a flowing waltz and Violetta Elvin's beautiful arm movements, 'like the gills of a transparent fish, conducting a submarine symphony'.[28] Fire, with Beryl Grey as its Queen, has swift changes of front, percussive movements, flickering hands, brilliance and athleticism. Air is a *pas de deux* in the grand manner of Petipa, and possibly amongst Ashton's best choreography. Fonteyn enters on the shoulders of Michael Somes, her regular partner, he being presented as a winged zephyr, supporting her in high and unusual lifts. She dances a swift variation that delights the audience.[29]

The ballet presents a whole series of hierarchies nested in each other: at the level of each elemental court scene, at the level of the whole ballet, and at the level of the Sadler's Wells Ballet and the place of this company in relation to the nation and the current royal moment. Each of the four elements is led by one of the company's classical ballerinas and her partner, one of the classical *danseurs* of the company, which in itself indicates the achievement of Sadler's Wells Ballet in having so many high ranking dancers at its disposal. There is, however, the sense that this must build to the *pas de deux* for Air, prima ballerina Margot Fonteyn and Michael Somes, he the most skilful and solicitous of balletic consorts. They are the most regal pair. In the retinues for each elemental 'court' are the regular *corps de ballet* dancers, gathering around their monarchs. Exceeding them in authority are the small ensemble dances, showing off the various characters and abilities of the soloists and principal dancers: Earth's *Pas de six,* Water's *Pas de trois,* Fire's *Pas de quatre,* and a sparky solo, Spirit of Fire, to show off Alexander Grant's fizzing, bravura technique. The apotheosis makes explicit the founding of this New Elizabethan Age as all the dancers face the rear of the stage where Queen Elizabeth I appears in all her Tudor majesty with orb and sceptre. A new figure comes to face her, with a huge and richly decorated crimson robe that flows across the stage towards the audience. We understand that Queen Elizabeth II pays homage to her Elizabethan forebear and now the ballet company pays homage to its new Queen. In this final symbolism, the serried ranks of Sadler's Wells Ballet at the Royal Opera House assert their position in relation to their ultimate Queen and her heritage, the dancers grouped as a coronet with Fonteyn as its diadem. In her scrapbook Monica Collingwood titles this picture, 'Crown Imperial' perhaps thinking of the 1937 Coronation march of this name by William Walton when the current Imperial State Crown was first used to crown the monarch. So *Homage to the Queen* ends by personifying the crown, the 'crowning glory', with which to symbolically crown the Queen, while declaring itself and its stars the essence and substance of that crown.

Monica amongst others has succumbed personally to Fonteyn's art

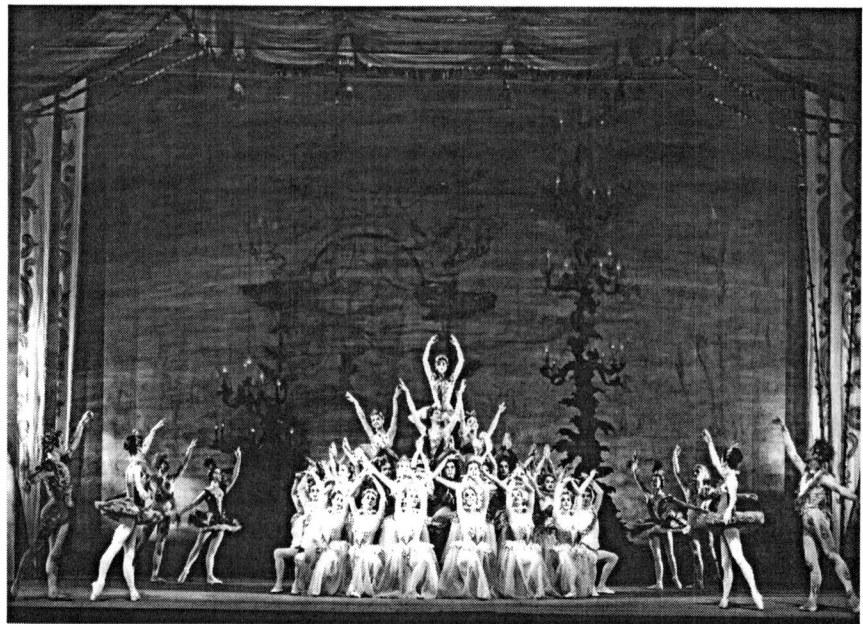

Sadler's Wells Ballet in the finale tableau of *Homage to the Queen* (chor. Ashton, 1953), with Margot Fonteyn at the pinnacle. Photo: ©Houston Rogers / V&A Images, Victoria and Albert Museum, London.

although many in the country know her only from the very fulsome press she receives. Associated with her queenly roles, she is 'Princess of Ballet'.[30] For Cyril Beaumont her pre-eminence in *The Sleeping Beauty* makes her 'Queen of Auroras'. She is a national treasure, an icon of a Britain that is still 'Great' despite the East/West clash that seems to be happening in a region where we have less political leverage: 'no ballerina in Free Europe or America can match her Princess Aurora or her Odette'.[31] Or she is 'Queen of the Dance'.[32] In the Coronation month's edition of *The Dancing Times*, with a new masthead, she is posed as Odette, the Swan Queen in *Swan Lake*, 'pre-eminently the dancer whose name future dance historians will associate with the Coronation Year of Queen Elizabeth'.[33]

* * * * *

On 8 June the Royal Coronation Gala takes place at the Royal Opera House with the premiere of Benjamin Britten's opera, *Gloriana*, dances choreographed by John Cranko. This is before an audience that includes both British and European royalty and those from further afield, the sultans, and Queen Salote of Tonga (a much loved presence in London throughout the Coronation season).[34] Of itself, this situation makes the gala a strange event, since so many, including the British contingent of the audience, do not normally go to opera and so many do not understand the modern genre in which Britten works. It is certainly a night when the splendour of the audience outdoes the stage. The Royal Box is fronted by cloth of gold and swags of flowers and has lights shaped into the figures of Saint George and Britannia. We are told (but as ordinary members of the audience we cannot verify) that the Royal Box ante-room is hung with gold silk and crystals and the Crush Bar, out of bounds to all except official guests, is similarly hung with silk and floral decorations.[35] Every jewelled tiara and every military decoration is on show. The royal household is all in attendance, gentlemen of the royal blood in court dress which includes the oddity of breeches and stockings with their tail coats. The glitter of the occasion is offset by a somewhat deadening formality, guardsmen on the stairs and foyers and Beefeaters from the Tower of London on guard in the auditorium. Britten's brief, to write an opera linking the new Queen to the first Elizabethan age, has resulted in a sordid story of Elizabeth and Essex and the regrets of an old Queen about her lost love. However psychologically revealing the topic, there are doubts about its appropriateness to an occasion hailing a new young Queen.

Dances happen in two scenes of Act Two. At Norwich the Queen is entertained by allegorical figures of Time and Concord with offerings by girls and men bringing flowers, fruit and fish. They dance with simple steps, to an unaccompanied chorus. In Scene Three there is a court ball at Whitehall in which dances of the period are represented: Pavane, Galliard, La Volta, Coranto.[36] While the ladies retire, 'to change their linen', a Morris dancer entertains the men.

The evening is not a success for much of the audience, who clap politely and frugally and are cold to the modernism of Britten's music. The evening drags on tediously.[37] Or else it seems such a superficial rendering of what we think of as a 'swashbuckling' age.[38] Even some who admire the opera find it does not excite an emotional connection.[39] Those on the ballet side of the Covent Garden disputes with opera reflect at this point on how right they were. *Homage* would have made such a better royal gala, rising to a wonderful apotheosis rather than the pathos of *Gloriana*.[40]

June 1953
17th : Uprising in East Berlin put down by Soviet tanks.
19th : Execution in USA of Communist Party members Julius and Ethel Rosenberg for passing atom bomb secrets to USSR.

From Bloomsbury to the Scala: trying to get hold of new things

I'm spending a few post-Coronation days in a new hotel in London that replaces the bombed-out range of houses on the south side of Tavistock Square in Bloomsbury. The Tavistock Hotel has an *art deco* theme, so appropriate since the hotel replaces the houses where Leonard and Virginia Woolf resided with their Hogarth Press between 1924 and 1939. While it's not up to the moment of our 1950s Festival Style of design, the hotel tries to evoke the atmosphere of a vibrant and carefree time between the Wars and it's decidedly twentieth century, not retrograde like so much at this Coronation time! I enjoy this frisson of being close to the Bloomsbury clans around these squares, but I'm looking for something much more up to date. I want the latest home designs. I want to see, or even buy, furnishings that have been promoted by the Festival of Britain. And I want to ask how this new idea of Commonwealth (at least new to the consciousness of ordinary people) can translate itself into a performance in a theatre.

So now I set off from my hotel, turn left and head off towards the Tottenham Court Road. I'm going to make a little diversion so I can pass through Chenies Street, where the Diaghilev Ballet used to rehearse in the Drill Hall. It's just an indulgence for the sake of dance history because what I really want is New!

Heal's on Tottenham Court Road is the 'mecca' for modern design. They weren't wrong, those people who said that Festival Style is 'all Heal's let loose' because Heal's designers were already selling domestic interiors with the vision of twentieth century modernity before the Festival made it popular. They have the Mansard Gallery on the top floor where they exhibit modern craft design like Danish stoneware pottery, and in the past the work of artists such as Picasso. The refinement of form to utility, simplicity and geometry is almost the natural language at Heal's. Now, with designers like Christopher Heal and Robin Day, they sell quality furniture that really captures postwar optimism. There's the contrast between pale wood and strong colours in walls and fabric. This year's 'Heal's Flat', exhibited at the Ideal Home Exhibition in March, and also here on their shop-floor, is just like that—jade green walls and orange carpet; splayed legs lifting furniture off the floor (use your new vacuum cleaner to get underneath!); boxy storage units with a minimum of surface decoration beyond the lustrous patina of the wood; subtle lighting from fitments based on the cone; Lucienne Day's curtain fabric, *Strata*, atmospheric with white ovals against a jade background. Heal's shows us how the coordination of design works to unclutter the mind as well as the house. You can shop to a budget. Their catalogue shows 'Two Rooms for Two People' for £395[41] and 'One Room for One Person' (the 'bedsit'), for £125.

I'm here to pick some of the new accessories: light fitments of cut-off conical shades on the barest of steel wire frames, and fabrics by Lucienne Day. She, more than any others, gives me a real vision of the future. *Calyx*, for the Homes and Gardens Pavilion, was the design that took the Festival by storm, the abstraction of flowers, leaves and stems into colour, shape and line. She also upholstered the seats in the Telecinema on the South Bank now the National Film Theatre. Now she is becoming emblematic of modern design. Having her curtain fabrics, some of which can be printed on cheaper material, is almost like having modern art at the centre of domestic life, even if we can't afford the full Heal's coordinated style transformation. Some of her new designs are quite wispy, like *Dandelion Clocks* of this year, with delicate drawing on an orange background. I prefer her dramatic ones: *Small Hours*, is a fantasy of night creatures on a black background (definitely not for a child's bedroom). *Spectators* strongly appeals to me as so relevant to Coronation year. Peg-like objects in white and orange on a dark background seem human: some have spectacles, and some have a single open round eye or a spiral like a spring where the eye should be. They all seem to be straining upwards, as if to see the procession passing by.[42]

I'm leaving Heal's, to cross Tottenham Court Road and walk down Tottenham Street (it runs alongside Goodge Street Station). Just on its corner with Charlotte Street I find the Scala Theatre, where I am interested to see a performance of Bulbul and His Oriental Ballet. Bulbul Chowdhury and his company are dancers from Pakistan. This is now only six years after partition and independence for the Indian sub-continent, and surely not one of us is unaware of the horrifying massacres that underlined that process. Just days ago the Pakistani prime minister rode in a carriage in the Coronation procession and acknowledged the Queen as Head of the Commonwealth but already there are talks of it becoming a republic like India, in Pakistan's case an 'Islamic Republic'. Whether Pakistan will stay in the Commonwealth is not decided. So Pakistan's culture and politics are interesting at the moment.

We have become so used to the dancers from India (Uday Shankar, Ram Gopal, Mrinalini Sarabhai) with their divine dances of the Hindu deities, their restraint and beauty. Gopal and his company were here just at the end of 1952 with, amongst other dances, *The Golden Eagle*, which is always associated with Gopal, and a *Bharata Natya Suite* of dances from the Tanjore temples of South India.[43] What can Muslim dances look like?

Bulbul's dances are often nationalist. We have *The Call*, in which dancing to drums and dancing with swords (for both male and female dancers) makes '[a] clarion call to the youth of the country to come forward and offer themselves for the cause of the motherland'. A dance drama about the man-made Bengal famine of 1943, *Lest We Forget*, is uncomfortable watching for those of us who reflect that it was under British administration. *Chandrasultana*, danced as a solo by Bulbul's wife, Afroza, is 'the Joan of Arc of the Moslem world' riding her horse to victory on the battlefield. There are also folk dances and some romantic duets, one inspired by the Persian poet Hafiz. *One Tavern Night* finishes the programme, with intrigue amongst slaves, dancing girls and poets. The overall impression of the programme is of secular lives, lived sometimes poetically and mythically, in a new country where memory and recent tragedy mix with a rich inherited culture. This has more affinity with Katherine Dunham's projection of life in black neighbourhoods than the elevated other-worldliness of Ram Gopal. Our London ballet critics are not very complimentary about Bulbul – 'sentimental, vulgar in expression, and limited in technique' says Richard Buckle.[44] Arnold Haskell puts him in 'the "wriggle school" of oriental dancing', which descends into monotony or comedy.[45] Some critics, perhaps ones who think of themselves as less authoritative about dance, have considered that there is something fresh and more worthy in what Bulbul is doing.[46] Yes, the performers shriek and writhe but there is a terrible story to be told.[47] Trying to tell the story of a new country born out of chaos is surely something to applaud in the second half of the twentieth century.

Buckle's dismissal of Bulbul's enterprise is strung onto the end of his reflections on the inability of dance to convey (for him at least) tragic themes, having just seen the new ballet of *Blood Wedding* by Alfred Rodrigues at Sadler's Wells and presumably finding it inadequate to the story by Lorca. Buckle is straining once more for that moment of revelation when the pure poetry in dance strikes deep into his soul (see page 58), all the more valuable, he thinks, because it cannot be predicted. He concludes that: 'Perhaps ballet must always disguise itself as something frivolous in order to have any effect.'[48] Can we agree with Buckle? In spite of all the pleasures and optimism of Coronation year, our world is still filled with public and private tragedies. Isn't dance enough of a serious art form to reflect them?

Ballets Jooss was at Sadler's Wells in April with a programme of the pre-war favourites with a few new dances.[49] In the 1930s, many people thought that the choreography of Jooss was the absolute pinnacle of presenting a serious theme making its grim point, but with a restraint that allows an aesthetic appreciation of dance, in this case European modern dance. In his latest season, *The Green Table* is shown again to be an excoriating essay in how the whims of politicians create an implacable calamity for innocent people. Although it dates from 1932, it never ages in its message. *Big City*, from the same time, does not seem nearly as relevant as it once did, with its top-hatted Libertine tempting away the young working class girl. There are other dances with slight stories set in olden times, with the generalised message about young people being able to make their own choices (*Pavane* and *Ball in Old Vienna*). Some comedy numbers lighten the message, including the new piece, *Night Train*.

A new work, *Journey in the Fog*, returns to the subject matter of *The Green Table*, now in the light of World War II experience. This 'journey' is for the postwar exile to find a way back to a real or symbolic home. Only a few years ago, in the austere 1940s, 'displaced persons' was a phrase we all knew (DPs for short). Europeans were on the move, finding a way home after concentration camps or prisoner-of-war camps, or simply trying to find a home that didn't transgress the new ethnic and political boundaries. Perhaps we do not want to remember those things any more. It's a shock to see the exiles in the Jooss ballet hopelessly and fatalistically accepting their lot when we know that reconstruction demands fortitude.[50] For many people now, the Jooss style and repertoire are retrograde and out of step with 'the tough and exhilarating nineteen-fifties'.[51] It's like the contrast between the sobriety of Jooss's favourite setting of black curtains and the vibrancy of Lucienne Day's fabrics. Should we dwell too much on the past? And is dance the right medium to do so? Lionel Bradley is critical of the Jooss repertoire but even more critical of the critics who dismiss it out of hand: 'for all its faults, [it] has something distinctive to say'. But that whole line of expression is now cut off as the city of Essen can no longer support the company.[52]

July
15th : Execution of John Christie for murders at 10 Rillington Place. Concerns that Timothy Evans had been wrongly executed previously.
27th: Armistice ends Korean War.

August
19th : Coup in Iran returns the Shah to power with help of Western powers. Oil production resumed.

From Covent Garden to Shaftesbury Avenue

The summer becomes so crowded with companies from different nations, with different styles and enthusiasms that it starts to be argued that London cannot provide good audiences for all of them. This is a somewhat more sober estimation of 'London: the dancing capital of the world' than we have heard about before. American Ballet Theatre takes up residence in the Royal Opera House in July, followed by the Danish Royal Ballet in August. Then Les Ballets de Paris de Roland Petit occupies the Stoll Theatre from late August. This happens alongside the usual company activity at Sadler's Wells Theatre and at the Royal Festival Hall where Festival Ballet has its Coronation Season. And unusually Ballet Rambert is able to have a short August season at Sadler's Wells Theatre instead of wearing itself out on provincial tours and dancing in outer London suburbs such as Hammersmith and Lewisham.

The Royal Danish Ballet has been a talking point since a gaggle of British critics was invited for their ballet festival in 1951.[53] And yet it seems they never performed abroad, secure in their home at Copenhagen's Royal Theatre, and a two hundred year ballet tradition. Compared to them, the companies of London and New York are latecomers indeed! Richard Buckle proselytised for a first ever visit to this country and it came to pass this year. The uniqueness of their repertoire and their dance style sets them apart. The uniformly high standard and virility of the male dancers is an eye-opener. The dancers are all comfortable in character dancing which gives some authenticity to national dancing in village scenes. They do large scale story ballets very well, especially the ones from their historic choreographer of the nineteenth century, August Bournonville. Here they present his *Napoli* (an Italian setting in three acts), *La Sylphide* (Scottish, in two acts) and *A Folktale* (Danish, three acts) all from the 1830s – 1850s with an extract from another, *Konservatoriet*, which demonstrates the Bournonville style and technique maintained by the company. They also have their own version of *Coppélia*, a three act ballet well known here but which they perform in their own inimitable style with a lightness and intelligence of staging that makes perfect sense of the story. More recent choreography and shorter works they also have, the most unique being *Qarrtsiluni*, a ballet about northern tribes awaiting the return of the sun after the arctic winter.

Now the Danish ability in telling these old-time stories puts some more life into a growing controversy. Is the full evening story ballet making a comeback? It was a nineteenth century innovation of Imperial Russia, but Michel Fokine, Diaghilev's first choreographer, dismissed the old style of which the multi-act ballet was a part, with its separation of story, told by mime, from plotless danced divertissement. And so the programme of short works in expressive movement style became the norm for Diaghilev's company and all those that set themselves in his mould. Though Diaghilev's revival of *Sleeping Beauty* (*The Sleeping Princess*) in London in 1921 was sneered at as old-fashioned by the modernist intelligentsia, these nineteenth-century ballets have become part of the scene for British audiences since the 1930s through the émigré stagings by Sergeyev. Perhaps nobody understood early on, how these would become so dominant. So, through the repertoires of Sadler's Wells Ballet and International Ballet, *Sleeping Beauty*, *Swan Lake*, *The Nutcracker* and *Coppélia* become increasingly popular along with the two act *Giselle*. Perhaps there is some notion that once you know a story, you can understand a dance. And the box office speaks for itself. At Covent Garden this year the mixed bill of three contrasting short works, a format that Diaghilev promoted for its modernity, has slower bookings than the full-length classics.[54]

There is possibly a trend developing towards newly choreographed full-length works in nineteenth-century style. Frederick Ashton made *Cinderella* in 1948 and last year (1952), *Sylvia*, both three act works on existing scenarios and music scores. With these two in the Sadler's Wells repertoire and renewed interest instigated by a new production of *Swan Lake* at Covent Garden, dance magazines are declaring the 'return' of the three act ballet.[55] Ivor Guest thinks that the three act story ballet returns as part of the post Diaghilev 'counter reformation' as the seat of power in ballet returns to the great opera houses like Paris and London as opposed to the itinerant companies. The demands of the multi-act spectacle, including realism in stage sets, can only satisfactorily be met in a settled organisation.[56]

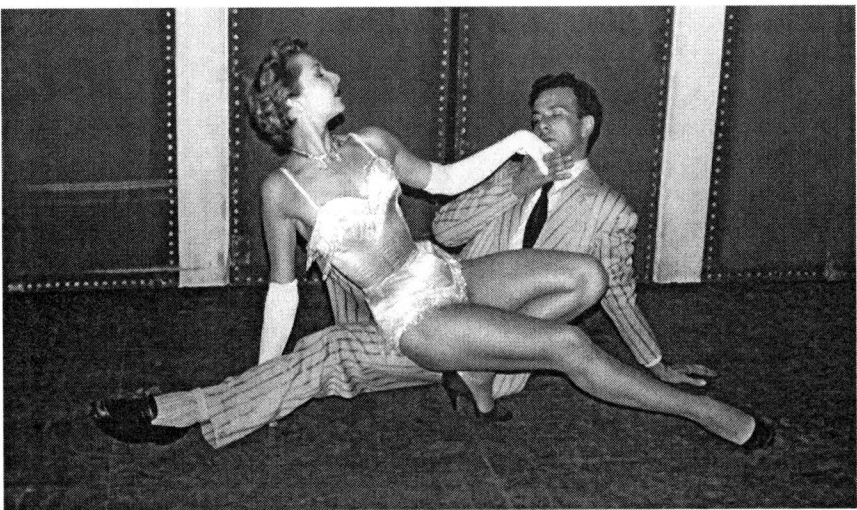

Roland Petit and Colette Marchand in *Ciné Bijou* (chor. Petit), Ballets de Paris at Stoll Theatre, August 1953. Photo: G.B.L. Wilson. © Royal Academy of Dance/ArenaPAL.

Is there a return to the three act ballet? Perhaps this is not one question but two. Audiences love the old three act ballets for their escapism and the way they test a favourite ballerina over the evening to develop her character throughout the story, and meet the technical demands of the big set-piece dances, solos and *pas de deux*. In this way Ashton's three-acters fit right into the nineteenth century mould (although *Cinderella* is to a twentieth century Prokofiev score, previously choreographed in Russia). Should these ballets be allowed to dominate the repertoire just because they are easy to understand and promote the star system? They seem to be quite opposite to the other trend in choreography of the last few years, in short plotless works like *Serenade* (Balanchine) and *Symphonic Variations* (Ashton) with their exquisite fusion of dancing and music, requiring no programme notes but rather an immersion in the moment of movement and music. Perhaps not every spectator is prepared to give that.

The other question is about the future of story ballets, whether they have one, two or three acts. If ballets are to tell stories, what kinds of stories should the story ballet be telling in this special year of 1953? The new three act ballets are fairy stories (*Cinderella*) and mythological (*Sylvia*). Festival Ballet is trying to jump on the bandwagon this year with *Alice in Wonderland* (in two acts), choreographed by Michael Charnley. Children's stories again! Isn't it possible to have gritty stories for adults of today, perhaps something like *Fall River Legend*, by Agnes de Mille presented this summer by American Ballet Theatre, exploring the case of the 1892 'axe murderer' Lizzie Borden. It's not a contemporary story but at least it aims for some psychological realism. A better example is *Ciné Bijou*, a contemporary ballet from Roland

Petit, performed this summer at the Stoll. Two single people go to watch a gangster movie and identify with the characters of a gangster and his moll in imagination. In the way of dream ballets they dance out the story of the film on the stage. It has passion and violence, smart suits and stiletto heels. But then, when the film ends, these people go their separate ways. How true to life![57]

Perhaps as the 'ballet boom' fades, stories will re-emerge for a public that cannot cope with more immersion in the wordless meanings of movement but the real question must be whether ballet or any other serious dance choreography can truthfully represent the lives of people today.

*   *   *   *   *

Ashton's *Sylvia* is mounted on a score and story from a ballet of 1876. Is that modernising or regressive? Clive Barnes considers that, in spite of its pre-Diaghilev origin and structure, Ashton's *Sylvia* is imbued with the expressivity of dancing inherited from Fokine and the new respect for purely classical dancing as shown in some recent pure dance works of Balanchine and Ashton.[58]

Sylvia, the female protagonist, has to carry the whole story through all three acts. Acolyte of the goddess Diana, she arrives in Act I, a woodland glade dominated by a shrine to Eros, heralded by a horn tune and her companions carrying the spoils of the hunt. They leap around in their helmets, brandishing their bows, looking single minded enough, but when the heat of the chase leaves them, the music and dancing are so sweet that we may wonder how they have the appetite for something so bloodthirsty. Devotee of her virginal goddess, Sylvia proudly rebuffs the love of the shepherd Aminta and mocks the statue of Eros. Aminta is struck by the arrow she intended for the statue, but this Eros is more alive than it appears. Craftily he lets off a love-inducing arrow at Sylvia who is hardly aware of what this means, even as she triumphs over the prostrate body of Aminta. Before the end of the scene, she has begun to feel love for Aminta but been abducted by the lustful Orion, a 'robber Khan'. Aminta is revived by a comic sorcerer, who we suspect to be Eros in disguise, and he is sent off in search of Sylvia.

In Act II she is a prisoner in Orion's grotto, listless and vulnerable at first but always capable of resistance, rejecting his advances and the constraints of his slaves and concubines. She is thrown around and pawed a lot but then conceives of a plan to get him and his crew intoxicated, so that she can escape. So she accepts a gold dress and assumes the oriental dance style of the Khan's palace. Her dance with finger cymbals is sexily enticing. But when her captors have collapsed in stupor she finds there is no way out! Eros comes to her aid, opening the cave for her escape.

The last act presents a festival before the temple of Diana, with dances from

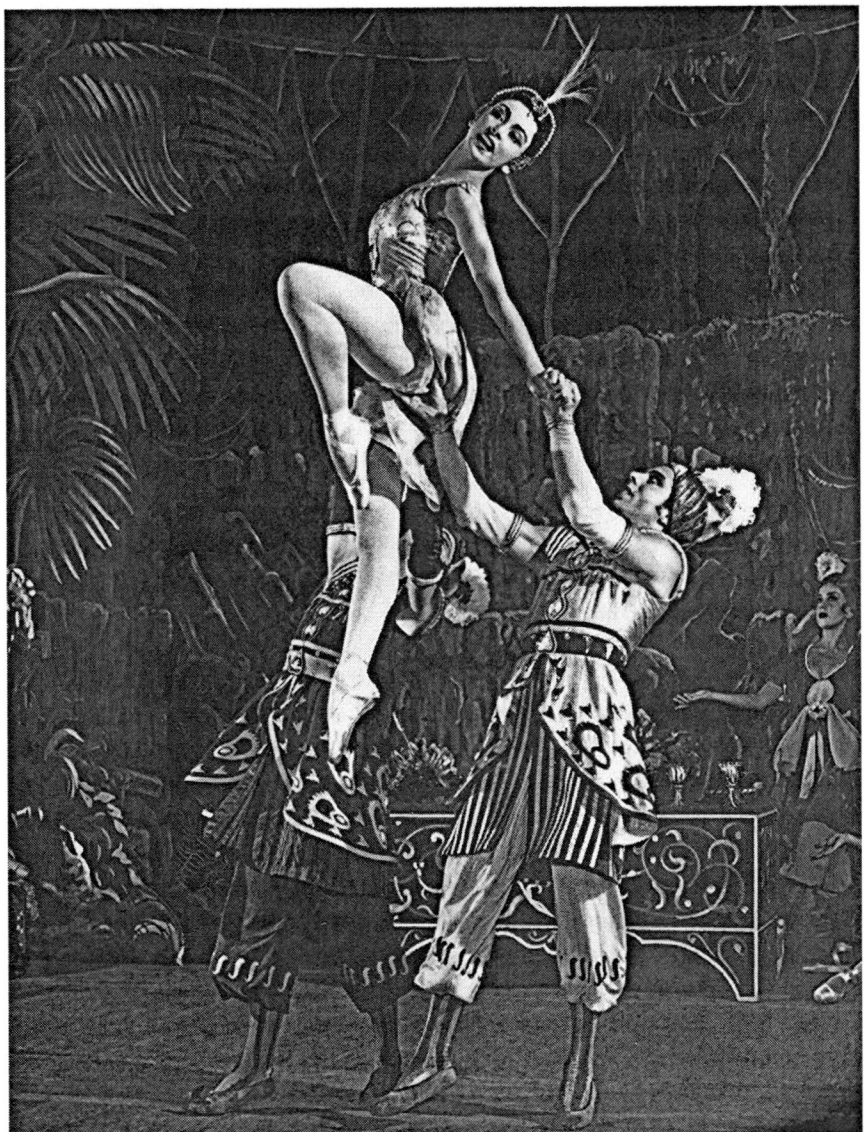

Margot Fonteyn as Sylvia, lifted by Peter Clegg and Brian Shaw as Slaves in Orion's Grotto, Act II of *Sylvia* (chor. Ashton,1952). Photo: © Felix Fonteyn. Courtesy of Mrs Phoebe Hookham.

Apollo and the Muses with other gods and goddesses and some cute goats. Aminta, is still in search of Sylvia having made no progress since Act I. How pathetic! When a ship brings Eros and Sylvia to the gathering, Aminta and Sylvia are finally united in a *pas de deux*, which is triumphant rather than erotic. Sylvia's solo variation to the infamous *pizzicato* (accompaniment to many a comedian's skit) is a triumph of choreographic intricacy and sparkling execution and her final entrance kneeling on Aminta's shoulder is magnificent. Yet Orion is also in pursuit. Unwisely he bangs on the temple door to be greeted by an enraged goddess Diana who dispatches him with an arrow, only to then turn her anger on the lovers, especially on Sylvia who should have been her virginal follower. Now Eros, with some magic of his own, causes a vision to appear, reminding Diana that she once herself fell in love with the shepherd Endymion. She can no longer refuse her blessing on the lovers and all is ironed out in celebration.[59]

Monica, who has a scrapbook devoted to *Sylvia*, sees the ballet in June during the Covent Garden Coronation season. She has seen it several times previously of course but it has renewed importance with Fonteyn, now fully recovered from her bout of diptheria, and on top form. She pronounces it 'Lovely, lovely, lovely'. As Clive Barnes eulogised when it premiered in 1952 (last year), it is most certainly Fonteyn's ballet:

> It exploits her every quality, her passion, her fierce imperiousness, her tenderness, her pathos, her womanliness, her bravura. It gives us Fonteyn triumphant, Fonteyn bewildered, Fonteyn exotic, Fonteyn pathetic, Fonteyn in excelsis.[60]

*   *   *   *   *

The straight walk to the Princes Theatre on Shaftesbury Avenue goes through the narrow Neal Street with its interesting courtyards. On the corner of Shaftesbury Avenue, is a shop advertising its valet service: 'My Business is Pressing'; 'I am Prepared to Dye for You'! Between it and the shop next door is the doorway of Nick's restaurant at 200 Shaftesbury Avenue, a favourite haunt of many dance fans and critics since it was the base for Carmen Amaya's gypsy family when she was performing at the Princes Theatre in 1948. John Betjeman deplores the fact that the windows of these pleasant Georgian houses are now covered in advertising hoardings.[61] Across from here, on a road island and somewhat separate from other theatreland venues of Shaftesbury Avenue, is the Princes Theatre. In 1921 and 1927 Diaghilev's Ballets Russes performed here.

Now, Walter Gore has the first season of his own company. Gore, it seems, has been around forever: working with Rambert and the Vic-Wells; working abroad; working in commercial theatre; and recently cropping up again in Ballet Workshop. He represents the other end of the ballet company spectrum from Covent Garden, with no full-length ballets and a repertoire built up in small (often transient) companies. The fifth generation of a theatrical family that travelled around working in temporary fit-ups, he moved from professional acting into dancing in his teenage years.[62] His programmes exploit the theatrical possibilities of an evening of short contrasting works. He has two main themes: light and amusing and dark

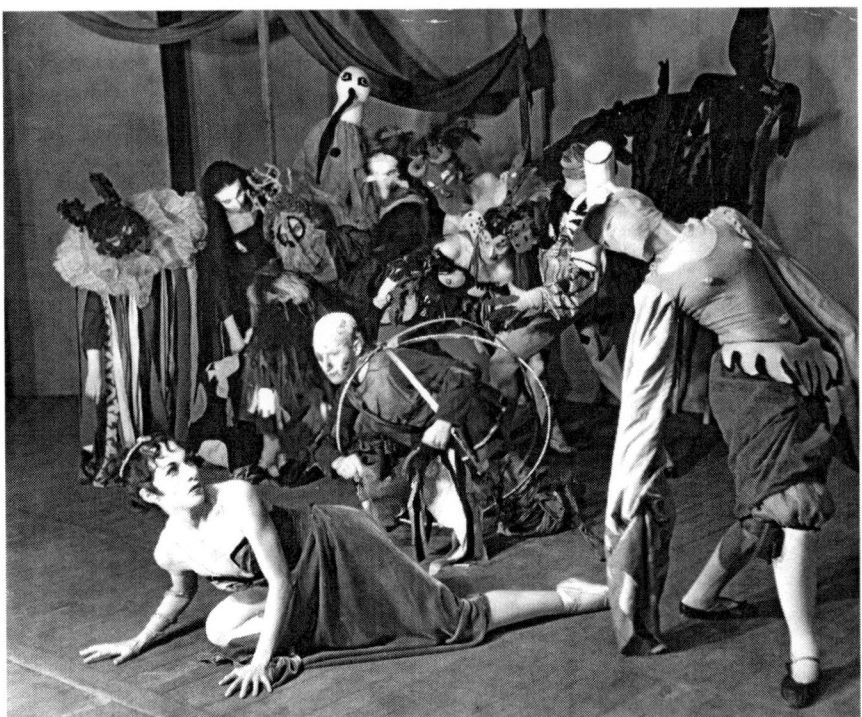

Paula Hinton (centre) tries to escape through the carnival crowd, in the title role of Walter Gore's ballet, *Antonia*. Photo: © Keystone Press Agency.

and dramatic. Titles like *Hoops* and *Light Fantastic* speak for themselves and we still laugh at *Peepshow* that was well received at Ballet Workshop last year (see p.79). *Street Games* is unusual, even for Gore, since it looks like an absolutely contemporary intrusion into the things children are doing now on the streets: 'Hopscotch', 'Rugger', 'Writing on the Wall', etc.

His dramatic themes are somewhat controversial, tending to melodrama. *Confessional*, in which a young woman faces death by the Spanish Inquisition, was especially associated with Sally Gilmour who danced it in her final performance with Ballet Rambert last year, before emigrating to Australia. Perhaps it could never be performed by anyone else. *Antonia* is another ballet with a horrifying theme, an unfaithful woman strangled by her lover. This season there is *Crucifix*, in which a young woman is burned for being a witch. The building tension bursts out with a terrifying scream coming from the girl as she burns and the curtain falls.[63] This is not frivolous ballet. Gore is a man of the theatre, which is so much wider than the conventions of opera house ballet.[64]

The question returns, if dances are to have stories, what stories can they tell? Many choreographers, like Bulbul, Jooss and Gore, wish to turn their attention to the horrors of life. Murders and persecutions are never far from our thoughts in the everyday of this postwar world, so it is appropriate, even necessary, for choreographers to reflect that. Perhaps Gore's twin themes properly reflect the knife edge between optimism and pessimism, or between facing the horrors and whistling in the dark. How to reflect the repugnant issues of the contemporary world without removing them to past centuries remains a problem for choreography in 1953.[65]

The walk from Covent Garden to the Princes Theatre is a walk from the high spots of subsidised ballet to the financial difficulties of unsubsidised touring companies; from the repertoire dominated by the classics to the personal artistic vision of a director-choreographer with new ideas on his mind. Can this company succeed? Since 1951 at least six small companies have gone out of business. [66]

September
13th : Sadler's Wells Ballet opens its third north American tour in New York.

October
19th: Old Bailey Trial of youths accused of a murder on Clapham Common. 'Teddy Boys' recognised as a social problem in London.

November
23rd : The Queen and Prince Philip embark on a six month tour of Commonwealth countries and colonies.

Down the Mall to Belgravia

Some of us may wish to take a nostalgic walk, remembering with satisfaction the pleasures of the year. The Mall is much quieter now. The Coronation decorations and stands have gone. Buckingham Palace flies only the Union Flag. The Royal Standard of blue, red and gold is not there since the Queen is on her travels. Further on, still moving west, past the grounds and gardens, it's the upmarket aristocratic housing of Belgravia, the smell of money and of power. Past Eaton Square and Belgrave Square, in the direction of Harrods, Lowndes Street is on the border of Knightsbridge. The houses are the same tall white stuccoed terraces although the addresses do not have the same cachet as Belgravia proper.

Margot Fonteyn recently moved into a top floor flat here, a 'penthouse'. The movement here from her previous address in Long Acre, right close to the Opera House, signals an advance in her status. It's not much of an exaggeration to make the analogy between her and the real Queen who is now nearly a neighbour, and of course, like Queen Elizabeth, Fonteyn is also currently delighting her subjects abroad as she tours America.

Before her departure, Fonteyn opened her new residence to the press. Reporting makes much of the colours of the new home. The dining room walls are red with white paint, recesses picked out with green paper; the living room has white walls with red soft furnishings. There is a hint of luxury:

a carpeted bathroom rather than a tiled one; expensive flock wallpaper in the bedroom; the drinks cabinet that can be filled from outside the room without the maid entering. There is not much to suggest that Fonteyn is wallowing in Festival Style. She has an outside veranda full of flower tubs, that 'continental' suggestion of outside living that the Festival promoted, and the 'so Festival' Venetian blinds in the bedroom but the furniture is a mixed collection of what she has picked up.[67] Truthfully, photographs of her home look more traditional than anything else: a landscape painting above the fireplace and candle sticks on the mantelpiece. Her copy of 'The Three Graces' statue by Canova lit in an alcove at the end of the corridor, seems so completely correct for a dancer whose art is based on harmonious and graceful proportions.

Fonteyn's position as *prima ballerina* is absolutely secure now. Her return to the full-length *Swan Lake* after two years in May was the moment for touching acclaim by the audience at Covent Garden, still totally at her command.[68] Lillian Moore acclaims her from New York, tempted to announce her 'the greatest ballerina in the world'. Her last performance there in *Sleeping Beauty* seemed to be totally secure in technique and yet danced with abandon.[69] She performs the *ballerina assoluta* on and off stage, now dressed by Dior in Paris or Cavanagh in London[70] but she is also admired for her lack of egotism in her work, her self-criticism, her strong ethic of self-improvement and loyalty to her company. None of her qualities – of musicality, technical finish, and expressiveness – is taken to an extreme. All in all, this niceness and good behaviour, loyalty, self-effacement and sheer hard work, can be seen as an icon of Britishness. This is the way the nation succeeds, just as she has.[71] Like the Queen, she provides a symbol for national identity. Her attributes of strength and imagination take us right back to the Lion and Unicorn pavilion in the South Bank Exhibition.[72] She reflects back to us the way we would like to be seen.

From the Aldwych to the Embankment: the River again

Aldwych on the Strand is like a semi-circular island of authority standing between two churches. The story of the building of Kingsway (see pages 37-38) is not complete without the story of Aldwych but its building up took even longer than Kingsway. Three major buildings stand there, circled by traffic but really centres of power. Australia House, opened in 1918, sits solidly at its eastern end, classical in style with rusticated ground floor arches and first floor columns. The apex on its triangular site appropriately faces east, surmounted high up by a huge bronze of Phoebus and the horses of the sun, almost like the figurehead of a ship pressing forward, riding down the Thames and crossing the ocean. India House, to its west, opened some ten years later, to take on part of the administration of Imperial India, now the High Commission of independent India. On its walls are coloured roundels with peacocks and other notions of the sub-continent's riches. Columns above the doorway are supported by elephant heads and topped by panthers. Between them is Bush House, its dramatic white stone portico shining like a beacon, facing the end of Kingsway. Although it looks so much like an imperial statement, it was built in the 1920s as offices for American companies, rather flatteringly with statues at its entrance symbolising the friendship of the English speaking peoples across the Atlantic. By 1953 it has acquired a new meaning, with the BBC World Service broadcasting from here since the war. The Cold War gives it a particular significance, with all the languages it broadcasts to Eastern European countries including Russia, broadcasts that are frequently blocked. So the Aldwych island now speaks *of* the Commonwealth and speaks *to* the world.

On 2 November my walk takes me from the busy and festive Aldwych, eastwards to the splendid gothic building of the Royal Courts of Justice. At this point the gateway to the City of London once stood, named Temple Bar, its position now marked by a monument topped with a griffin. I go no further into the City but turn towards the river, through the lanes and courtyards of the fraternities of lawyers inhabiting two of those ancient Inns of Court, Inner and Middle Temple. Tonight there is to be a ballet performance in Middle Temple Hall, under the Elizabethan hammer beam roof. This area suffered badly from war damage. The Hall was hit by a parachute mine destroying the screen and gallery which were reassembled, now completely restored, and the performance is to raise funds towards restoration and upkeep of the Temple Church which had severe damage from incendiaries. The long history of this corner of London goes back to the Knights Templar of the Crusades who built the church. Subsequently, the legal institutions of Middle and Inner Temple were erected on Templar land. When this Hall was built in the sixteenth century it became the scene of revels, misrules, masques and dancing from the members and professional companies, including (it is thought) the first performance of Shakespeare's *Twelfth Night* in 1602. Our current London theatres and those 'theatres' of London's political power like Kingsway, Aldwych and the Mall, are mere children in comparison to the length of history saturating this Hall. While our lawyers of the 1950s cannot always be expected to foxtrot or waltz competently,[73] those of the sixteenth and seventeenth centuries were required to dance the 'Old Measures' (almains, brawles, corantos, pavins and galliards)[74] during ceremonies and entertainments.

Middle Temple Hall in 1953 is a centre for its members, for daily meals, ceremonies and plays. For the first time here there will be a ballet performance. At the western end of the Hall, a black box proscenium stage has been set up, and Ballet Rambert performs for a select and paying audience (one to four guineas), the guest of honour being Queen Elizabeth the Queen Mother, who has had the honorary position of Royal Bencher since 1944. This is a welcome idea for everyone. The Treasurer (head of Middle Temple) is a friend of Marie Rambert and the Queen Mother has taken an interest in her work since the early days of the company, making a point nowadays of speaking to Rambert when their paths cross at galas.[75] Tonight Rambert is on hand amongst guests in an anteroom before the performance.[76] Conditions in the Hall are not ideal for the company with no room for scenery and necessarily an *ad hoc* lighting set-up. Music is provided by two pianos and a string quartet. Yet the atmosphere of the Hall, its reconstruction a positive story of postwar recovery, and the glamour of the royal occasion, bring together ideas that have occupied us in Coronation year.

The programme condenses a history of ballet and of the company. Tchaikovsky's music and the nineteenth-century Russian classics are represented by the *grand pas de deux* from *The Nutcracker* and *Swan Lake*, Act II. Then, Andrée Howard's *Death and the Maiden* to Schubert's music and Ashton's ever popular *Façade* with music by William Walton, remind us how vibrant was the choreographic culture of Rambert's little band, the Ballet Club, in London in the 1930s. *Death and the Maiden* is particularly noted as working well with the lighting, which creates *chiaroscura* effects in the depths of the stage. Where do we go from here? The new, popular work *Movimientos* by Michael Charnley, which started life last year in Ballet Workshop, is persuasive about blending modern dance and musical theatre techniques with the balletic ones of the Rambert dancers, more so with the choreographer here as guest artist.[77] Between the panelled walls, underneath the array of massive oak beams and finials, with portraits looking down, it seems that the story as told tonight, balletically, musically and architecturally, is of smooth progress from past to present to future.

*　*　*　*　*

Still vibrating from the modern, Latin rhythms of *Movimientos*, and the 1920s Tango from *Façade*, I walk a little way to the Victoria Embankment on the favoured north bank, and look on the Thames again. Up to the mid-nineteenth century, the water flowed right up to the Water Gate entrance of the Middle Temple Hall, across the land now taken up by road, embankment, gardens and later Temple buildings. Underneath my feet are the engineering achievements of that century – sewers and tube trains. Our recent history is preserved on the Embankment wall: a World War II convoy escort ship, HMS Wellington, is now moored here, near the extensive and poignant Submariners Memorial. The electric standards bordering the Embankment, shafts curled around with dolphin forms, cast dim traces across the oily water. Vaguely illuminated vessels are still working, puttering and smoking in the cold air. The *Ars Magna* of London again.

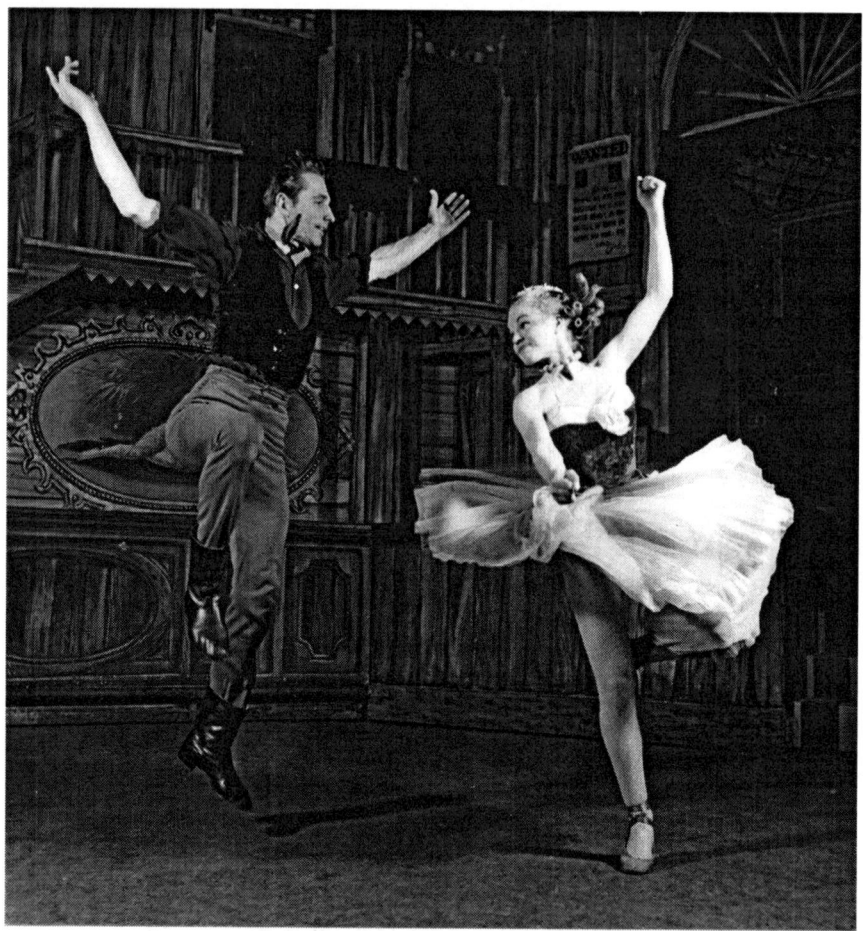

Veit Bethke and Sheila O'Neill dancing in the London production of *Paint Your Wagon*, 1953. Photo: © John Chillingworth/Getty Images.

As I walk towards Waterloo Bridge and the Station, the city sounds open up the space to feel other places, other venues and other dances. While our ballet companies are all currently touring abroad or in the provinces (including Ballet Rambert which has to pack up tonight and head for Cambridge), London still gives us dances. Tonight at the Stoll, the show is *Braziliana*, electrifying the audience with its finale, 'Festival in Rio'. At the Theatre Royal, Drury Lane, *The King and I*, is the latest American musical, with its perfectly crafted little ballet choreographed by Jerome Robbins, 'The Small House of Uncle Thomas', a Siamese-styled version of Harriet Beecher Stowe's *Uncle Tom's Cabin*. True to the new structure of musical theatre choreography, it's a device paralleling the emotional plotline of a runaway girl. At the Coliseum, the Queen is attending the Royal Variety Performance. Dance acts include Sheila O'Neill and Veit Bethke performing their dance from *Paint Your Wagon*. Sometimes referred to as 'The Pony Ballet' or the 'Skipping Rope Dance', it was the only thing approved of by many of our critics.[78] The forty Tiller Girls, the high-kicking squad rivalling New York's Rockettes, is there as well, and no doubt receiving huge applause. These and other audiences swell the pedestrian traffic on my walk.

Right by the north entrance of Waterloo Bridge, the now sooty Somerset House, full of government offices, no longer rises dramatically from the water as in the eighteenth and early nineteenth centuries, but still represents tradition and power. Over on the South Bank, the Royal Festival Hall is now looking isolated, but nevertheless is a beacon of a new kind of theatre and represents some sense of renewal. Dance furnishes so many delights. The small screen of the television and even the big screen of the cinema give very little in comparison to live theatre, and so must remain a passing fad for ballet performances. Tonight I have had re-acquaintance with old favourites – *Swan Lake*, *Death and the Maiden* and *Façade* and I have seen the promise of the future. Michael Charnley is just one of those choreographers of today with advanced ideas, the youngsters to succeed Frederick Ashton's generation. We have the appetite for more of Charnley's South American rhythms; more of John Cranko's comedies; and more of Jack Carter's atmospheric dances with unsettling hints of a Proustian story.[79]

The Sunday Times carried a rehearsal photograph on its front page yesterday, *Swan Lake* Act II in the Middle Temple Hall, right next to a headline, 'East Germans Report Big Revolt Plot'.[80] Even our most cherished experiences of pure aesthetic delight, it seems, must be contaminated by the international situation, the East/West split and Soviet paranoia over its hold on East Germany. Dance, like an international language, should be above political rifts. In a few days, at the Scala Theatre, London will see its first Soviet dancers in person: a trio from the Piatnitsky folk dance ensemble, Georgi Farmanyants from the Bolshoi Ballet, Alla Shelest and Konstantin Shatilov from the Kirov Ballet, and a dancer from the Uzbek State Theatre.[81]

While the trains rattle and smoke their last journeys of the night, tomorrow holds promise of yet more years of London as the dance capital of the world.

Notes

1   Available from British Pathé archive, http://www.britishpathe.com/video/queen-sees-ideal-homes-1 accessed February 2013.
2   'The Ann Temple House', *Daily Mail Ideal Home Exhibition Catalogue and Review*, Olympia March 1953, p.99.
3   Statistics on average earnings historically vary considerably across sources. The range for average weekly earnings in 1953 seems to be £9-£12 which puts yearly average income approximately in the range £400-£600.
4   Janet Rowson Davies is the detailed documenter of BBC dance transmission from 1932-1959. See articles in the bibliography for citations relevant to the period of this book.
5   This performance of *Les Sylphides*, produced by Christian Simpson, is one of the very few early television ballets preserved on videotape, available to view at the National Film Archive of the British Film Institute and also now on DVD.
6   The Coronation Souvenir Programme opens with the symbols of the seven previous Empire colonies which have now become autonomous and equal Commonwealth Member Countries with Britain. At this point, India is the only one of them that is a republic, acknowledging the Queen as Head of the Commonwealth but not as Head of State. (Pakistan soon follows this arrangement). Fifty other overseas British administrations of various types are listed.
7   Julie Kavanagh (1996) *Secret Muses: The Life of Frederick Ashton*, p.408.
8   'Festival Pleasure Gardens' Third Season: Coronation Features', *The Times*, 15 May 1953, p.3.
9   I am aware that I am stretching the term *prima ballerina assoluta* which is an official accolade, very rarely given. My use of the term reflects the occasional usage for Markova and Fonteyn in the dance press of the period. Fonteyn did not officially receive the title until she was on the point of retiring from dancing in 1979. See: Peter Williams, 'The Crown of Supremacy', *Dance and Dancers*, June 1953, p.5.
10 Taglioni appeared at the King's Theatre (named Her Majesty's from late twentieth century) in *La Bayadère* (chor. Deshayes, mus. Auber), in 1831. It appears that the 1832 sketch by Princess Victoria is a good copy of the famous lithograph by Chalon of Taglioni in that ballet. Duvernay appeared at Drury Lane in 1833 in *The Sleeping Beauty*, based on the Paris Opera's version (chor. Jean Aumer, mus. Hérold)
11 Jasper Howlett, 'Queen Victoria and the Ballet', *Ballet*, March-April, 1947, pp.49-51. The dolls are currently in the Museum of London. The journals and sketchbooks are now available online: http://www.queenvictoriasjournals.org
12 Sadly, the Queen thought Taglioni, 'too old now to give real pleasure', although she was also 'wonderful'. For her, Grisi was the victor. Queen Victoria's Journals, 17 July 1845.
13 The collection is held in the Theatre Museum Collection at the Victoria and Albert Museum, London. See: Sarah Woodcock, 'Margaret Rolfe's Memoirs of Marie Taglioni: Part 1', *Dance Research*, v.7, no.1, Spring 1989, pp.3-19.
14 The Teck family lived in the royal grace-and-favour residence, White Lodge, in Richmond Park. White Lodge became the Sadler's Wells (Royal) Ballet Lower School in 1955.
15 James Pope-Hennessy (1959) *Queen Mary*, London: Unwin Hyman, p.77.
16 These anecdotes occur in various sources with minor differences and might be embellishments on the same incident: Ivor Guest (1958) *Adeline Genée: a lifetime of ballet under six reigns, based on the personal reminiscences of Dame Adeline Genée-Isitt*,

D.B.E, London: A & C Black, pp.192-193; Julian Braunsweg(1973), p.123; Anton Dolin, 'Royal Patrons of the Ballet', *Dance and Dancers*, June 1953, pp.11-12.

17 Woodcock, 'Margaret Rolfe's Memoirs of Marie Taglioni: Part 1', *Dance Research*, v.7, no.1, Spring 1989, pp.11-12.

18 Anton Dolin, 'Royal Patrons of the Ballet', *Dance and Dancers*, June 1953, p.11.

19 Her Highness Princess Marie Louise (1956) *Memories of Six Reigns*, p.40.

20 Julian Braunsweg (1973), *Ballet Scandals*, p.125.

21 Anton Dolin, 'Royal Patrons of the Ballet', *Dance and Dancers*, June 1953, p.12.

22 'Diamonds are worn at Royal Night Out', unidentified press cutting in Monica Collingwood Collection, Scrapbook (Tower Bridge No.1). The occasion is the Royal Gala for the premiere of Frederick Ashton's ballet, *Tiresias*, 9 July 1951.

23 William Shakespeare, *The Tempest*, Caliban, Act 3, Scene 2.

24 'Sadler's Wells Ballet: "Homage to the Queen"' *The Times*, 3 June 1953, p.20. It can only be coincidence that the same quotation, including the preceding 'Be not afeard', began the 2012 London Olympics Opening Ceremony, *Isles of Wonder*, spoken by the actor Kenneth Branagh in the character of Isambard Kingdom Brunel. In both cases the quotation has appropriate national, historical and spectacular connotations.

25 Norman Lebrecht (2000) p.141 describes infighting between ballet and opera interests over the honour of presenting the gala for the new Queen.

26 Peter Williams, 'Royal Parallel', *Dance and Dancers*, June 1953, pp.7-10; July 1953, pp.5-6; August 1953, pp.7-8; September 1953, pp. 7-8.

27 'Broadcast by the Queen: Inspiration of Loyalty', *The Times*, 3 June 1953, p.12.

28 Richard Buckle, 'Ballet', *The Observer*, 7 June 1953, p.12.

29 My description of *Homage to the Queen* is based on the following sources: Barnes, Hunt and Williams, 'Homage to the Queen', *Dance and Dancers*, August 1953, pp.12-13; Cyril Beaumont, 'Homage to the Queen', *Sunday Times*, 7 June 1953; Lionel Bradley, Ballet Bulletins, 2 June 1953; Richard Buckle, 'Ballet', *The Observer*, 7 June 1953, p.12; Julie Kavanagh (1996) *Secret Muses*, pp.408-409; 'Homage to the Queen', *The Dancing Times*, July 1953, pp.597-598.

30 'Princess of Ballet: Godfrey Winn introduces Margot Fonteyn', cutting in Monica Collingwood scrapbook, Fonteyn No. 1, probably late 1940s.

31 'Portrait Gallery: Margot Fonteyn', *Sunday Times*, 18 February 1951, cutting in Monica Collingwood scrapbook, Fonteyn No. 1.

32 'News Review', 9 March 1950, cutting in Monica Collingwood scrapbook, 'Dance Magazine'.

33 The Sitter Out, *The Dancing Times*, June 1953, p.529.

34 The atmosphere of the gala opening of the event, with arrivals and greetings at the Royal Opera House is captured in the British Pathé online archive, *The Crowning Year, Review of 1953*, and in particular in extensive unused footage in *Royal Opera Night 1953*.

35 'Queen at Covent Garden: Brilliant Premiere for "Gloriana"', *The Stage*, 11 June 1953, p.11.

36 Lionel Bradley, Ballet Bulletins, 11 June 1953; 30 June; 4, 11 July.

37 Beverley Baxter, MP, 'Covent Garden's Strangest Night: Mr Britten puts a chill on Merrie England', press cutting in Royal Opera House file, V&A Theatre Museum Collection.

38 Richard Capell, 'Reflections on "Gloriana": Limits of Medium', *Evening Standard*, 9 June 1953, press cutting in Royal Opera House file, V&A Theatre Museum Collection.

39 Eric Blom, 'Gloriana', *The Observer*, 14 June 1953, press cutting in Monica Collingwood Collection.

40 Peter Williams, 'Glory, Glory, Gloriana', *Dance and Dancers*, July 1953, p.3. The view from 2013 is somewhat different. While Ashton's choreography for *Homage* is mainly lost, Britten's opera will receive a revival in 2013, its 60th anniversary. It is an open question as to what factors have brought about this result, which must include the fact that dances were not regularly recorded in notation or in film at this time.

41 See this chapter, note 3, for comparison with annual average earnings.

42 My descriptions of Heal's and Lucienne Day's design is based upon: V&A Archive of Art and Design (Blythe House), Heal's 1953 file, AAD/1994/16/2857, and Lesley Jackson (2001) *Robin and Lucienne Day : Pioneers of Contemporary Design.*

43 Peter Williams, 'Ram Gopal', *Dance and Dancers*, January 1953, p.23.

44 Richard Buckle, 'Boundaries of Ballet', *The Observer*, 21 June, 1953, p.13.

45 '"Bulbul" and His Oriental Ballet: Scala Theatre' (1954), *Ballet Annual: Eighth issue*, p.44. See also 'Bulbul's Oriental Ballet', *The Dancing Times*, July 1953, p. 615.

46 For example: 'Scala Theatre: Ballet from Pakistan', *The Times*, 16 June 1953, p.10; 'Our London Correspondence', *The Manchester Guardian*, 17 June 1953, p.6.

47 Bulbul Chowdhury (1919-1954) is considered one of the founders of modern dance in Bangladesh, as East Pakistan became after the civil war of 1971. He was influenced by Rabindranath Tagore and Uday Shankar. The Bulbul Latikala Academy was set up in Dhaka after his death. See *Banglapedia: National Encyclopedia of Bangladesh*, http://www.banglapedia.org/HT/D_0019.HTM, accessed February 2013.

48 Buckle, 'Boundaries of Ballet', *The Observer*, 21 June, 1953, p.13.

49 Following an escape from Essen when Hitler became Chancellor of Germany in 1933, this modern dance company and school was given a base in England at Dartington Hall, Devon. Following the internment of Jooss and some of his colleagues in 1940, the company was able to reform in Cambridge in 1943 and tour Britain and the continent until 1947, when Arts Council funding ceased. Jooss returned to Essen in 1949.

50 'Ballets Jooss in London', *The Dancing Times*, May 1953, pp.470-471.

51 Dorothy Pratt, 'Ballets Jooss at Sadler's Wells', *Ballet Today*, May 1953, p.5.

52 Lionel Bradley, Ballet Bulletins, 28 April 1953. The continued life of *The Green Table* in many subsequent mountings on companies in Europe and America testifies to its quality and longevity. Bradley would have approved!

53 Buckle, (1953) *Adventures of a Ballet Critic*, pp.236-246.

54 Peter Williams, 'Full-Length Works Only?', *Dance and Dancers*, February 1953, p.5.

55 John Percival, 'Has the full-length ballet come to stay? Ashton points the way', *Dance and Dancers*, April 1953, p.10; Pamela Price, 'Will it be a "3A" future?', *Ballet Today*, August 1953, p.23.

56 'Four Opinions of Ashton's "Sylvia": Ivor Guest: "Sylvia" and the Future', *Ballet*, October 1952, pp.16-17.

57 There was a colour spread in *Picture Post*, 20 June 1953.

58 Clive Barnes, '*Sylvia*: New version of old classic', *Dance and Dancers*, November 1952, pp.12-15.

59 I base my description on contemporary accounts including Lionel Bradley, 3 September 1952. Video material includes: *Sylvia from the Royal Opera House, Covent Garden*, with Darcey Bussell and Roberto Bolle, transmitted by BBC 2, 25 December 2005; archive footage 1963, with Doreen Wells and John Gilpin, Royal Opera House Archive. Note that the boat that brings Sylvia to Act III did not appear at the end of Act II in the original production as it does in the 2004 revival.

60 Clive Barnes, '*Sylvia*: New version of old classic', *Dance and Dancers*, November 1952, p.14.

61 John Betjeman, 'Ballet-Goer's London Guide: 6', *Ballet*, May 1952, pp.30-31. With sketch by David Thomas.

62 Peter Williams, 'Theatre in the blood', *Dance and Dancers*, May 1953, pp.8-9.

63 Clive Barnes. 'New Ballets by Walter Gore: Crucifix', *Dance and Dancers*, November 1953, p.14.

64 Wendy Hilton, who performed in the pre-London tour of this short-lived company, was deeply disappointed in Gore's directorial and administrative ability (Wendy Hilton and Susan Bindig, 2010, *Wendy Hilton: A Life in Baroque Music and Dance*, pp.50-53). This autobiography gives a vivid account of the life of a 'jobbing' dancer in the 1950s.

65 In March 1954 Michael Holmes presented, *Common Ground* at Ballet Workshop, based on the murder on Clapham Common and in contemporary dress. It was not considered a success but there were also some criticisms that the theme was inappropriately close to real life.

66 It is quite difficult to track some of the smaller companies, which might simply work for isolated seasons, however the following are better documented: Ballet Nègres (1946-52); Ambassador Ballet (1949-51); London Theatre Ballet (1951); Empire Ballet (1949-52); Ballet Legat (1952); The New-Ballet Company (1952). The Walter Gore Ballet did not last beyond 1953 and International Ballet was forced to close down at the end of the year because it could not obtain Arts Council Funding.

67 Barbara Wace, 'Top of the Tree. 3: Margot Fonteyn', *Everywoman*, November 1953, pp. 40, 42-43, 85, 87. Some of the same material appeared in: Gordon Beckles, 'Margot Fonteyn', *Illustrated*, 20 February 1954.

68 Peter Williams, 'Fonteyn in the Lake', *Dance and Dancers*, June 1953, p. 26; Dorothy Pratt, 'Fonteyn in Lac des Cygnes', *Ballet Today*, June 1953, pp.17, 19.

69 Lillian Moore, 'By All Means – Fonteyn: New York Notes', *The Dancing Times*, December 1953, pp.132-134.

70 Wace, 'Top of the Tree. 3: Margot Fonteyn', *Everywoman*, November 1953,p. 85.

71 Peter Williams, 'The Fonteyn Way is typical of the British way', *Dance and Dancers*, December 1954, pp.12-13. See also: Barbara Wace, 'Top of the Tree.3: Margot Fonteyn', *Everywoman*, November 1953, pp. 40, 42-43, 85, 87; Wace '"My favourite role – I have none" – says Margot Fonteyn', *Ballet Today*, June 1953, pp.4, 5, 22.

72 Although this is not the place for a full scale examination of why Fonteyn was being written into this symbolic role, I consider it at least feasible as a starting point to consider how she was promoted as a figure of consensus validating the worth of state subsidy of the arts in establishing a new role for Britain in the world. The traits recognised by the Lion and Unicorn and press reports on Fonteyn, particularly reasonableness, lack of fanaticism and tendency to fantasy, are also identified in: Nikolaus Pevsner (1956) *The Englishness of English Art*, London: The Architectural Press [developed from previous writings in 1950s including 1955 Reith Lecture].

73 Mercutio, 'Miscellany: Temple Dancers', *The Manchester Guardian*, 7 November 1953, p.3.

74 James Cunningham (1965) *Dancing in the Inns of Court*, London: Jordan and Sons. This publication has been critiqued and corrected including from: David Wilson (1986-7) 'Dancing in the Inns of Court' *Historical Dance*, vol. 2, no.5, pp.3-16; Wilson (1994) 'The Old Measures and the Inns of Court: a Note', *Historical Dance*, vol. 3, no.3, p.24. The latter are available on the website of the Dolmetsch Historical Dance Society.

75 'Curtain Up: Queen Mother loves ballet', *Dance and Dancers*, December 1953, p.20.

76 Organisational details of the performance are preserved in Middle Temple Archive,

File NT.7/ROY/54, *Rambert Ballet in Hall, Monday 2nd November 1953.*

77 'For the Queen Mother', *Dance and Dancers*, December 1953, p.27; 'Ballet in Middle Temple: A Royal Occasion', *The Times*, 3 November 1953, p.3. I acknowledge the help of Lesley Whitelaw, archivist of Middle Temple, in contextualising this performance.

78 Choreography was by Agnes de Mille. See: Peter Williams, 'Ballet in Musicals: Paint Your Wagon', *Dance and Dancers*, April 1953, p.13. Review in *The Sunday Times* 15 February 1953 states: 'For a quarter of an hour this vulgarity is taken hold of by a young dancer, Sheila O'Neill, and intensified and transfigured. Desire loses its crudity, and in her pale, rapt face becomes a thing for pity and compassion.'

79 In 1953 Frank Jackson picked out these three for his book *They Make Tomorrow's Ballet*. Of the three, Charnley's career was to stall; Cranko went on to international fame as choreographer/ director of the Stuttgart Ballet (and not mainly recognised for choreographic comedies), although he died tragically young; and Carter's subsequent work, both abroad and for major British companies such as Royal and Festival ballets, was often sporadic, although it included some arguable masterpieces such as *Witch Boy* (1956).

80 *The Sunday Times*, 1 November 1953, p.1.

81 The political underpinning of these visits gradually became obvious. See: Larraine Nicholas, 'Fellow Travellers: Dance and British Cold War Politics in the Early 1950s', *Dance Research*, v.19, no.2, Winter 2001, pp.83-105.

SELECTIVE BIBLIOGRAPHY

See endnotes for references to journals and other sources.

Banham, Mary and Bevis Hillier eds. (1976) *A Tonic to the Nation: The Festival of Britain 1951*, London: Thames and Hudson.

Braunsweg, Julian (1973) *Ballet Scandals*, London: George Allen and Unwin.

Buckle, Richard ed. (1949) *Katherine Dunham: Her Dancers, Singers and Musicians*, London: Ballet Publications.

Buckle, Richard (1953) *The Adventures of a Ballet Critic*, London: Cresset Press.

Certeau, Michel de (1984), *The Practice of Everyday Life*, trans. Steven Rendall, Berkeley: University of California Press.

Coverley, Merlin (2006) *Psychogeography*, Harpenden: Pocket Essentials.

Daubeny, Peter (1971) *My World of Theatre*, London: Jonathan Cape.

Dolin, Anton (1953) *Markova: Her Life and Art*, London: W.H. Allen.

Dolin, Anton (1960) *Autobiography*, London: Oldbourne Books.

Festival of Britain (1951) *The Festival of Britain 1951: the Official Book of the Festival of Britain*, London: HMSO.

Festival of Britain (1951) *Festival Pleasure Gardens: Official Guide*, London: HMSO.

Franks, A.H. (1954) *Twentieth Century Ballet*, Westport, CT: Greenwood Press.

Franks, A.H. ed. (1955) *Ballet: A Decade of Endeavour*, London: Burke.

Gibbon, Monk (1951) *The Tales of Hoffmann*, London: Saturn Press.

Haskell, Arnold (1951) *In His True Centre: An Interim Autobiography*, London, Adam and Charles Black.

Hennessy, Peter (1993) *Never Again: Britain 1945-51*, London: Vintage.

Hennessy, Peter (2006) *Having it So Good*, London: Allen Lane.

Hewison, Robert (1988) *In Anger: Culture in the Cold War, 1945-60*, revised edition, London: Methuen.

Hewison, Robert (1995) *Culture and Consensus: England, Art and Politics since 1940*, London: Methuen.

High, David (1985) *The First Hundred Years: The Story of the Empire, Leicester Square*, Woldingham, Surrey: David High.

Hillier, Bevis (1975) *Austerity/Binge*, London: Studio Vista.

Hillier, Bevis (1983) *The Style of the Century: 1900-1980*, London: The Herbert Press.

Hilton, Wendy and Susan Bindig (2010) *Wendy Hilton: A Life in Baroque Dance and Music*, Hillsdale, NY: Pendragon Press.

Ingold, Tim (2007) *Lines: A Brief History*, London: Routledge.

Ingold, Tim (2011) *Being Alive: Essays on Movement, Knowledge and Description*, London: Routledge.

Jackson, Frank (1953) *They Make Tomorrow's Ballet*, London: Meridian Books.

Jackson, Lesley (2001) *Robin and Lucienne Day : Pioneers of Contemporary Design*, London: Mitchell Beazley.

Kavanagh, Julie (1996) *Secret Muses: The Life of Frederick Ashton*, London: Faber and Faber.

Kynaston, David (2007) *Austerity Britain, 1945-51*, London: Bloomsbury.

Lebrecht, Norman (2000) *Covent Garden: The Untold Story*, London: Simon and Schuster.

Leonard, Maurice (1995) *Markova the Legend*, London: Hodder and Stoughton.

Machen, Arthur (1988) *The Collected Arthur Machen*, Christopher Palmer, ed., London: Duckworth.

Marie Louise, H.H. (1956) *Memories of Six Reigns*, London: Evans Brothers Ltd.

MacInnes, Colin (1966) *England, Half English: A Polyphoto of the Fifties*, second edition, Harmondsworth: Penguin, first published 1961.

Moynahan, Brian (2007) *Looking Back at Britain: Road to Recovery – 1950s*, London: The Reader's Digest Association Ltd.

Nicholson, Geoff (2010) *The Lost Art of Walking: The History, Science, Philosophy, Literature, Theory and Practice of Pedestrianism*, Chelmsford: Harbour Books.

Pope-Hennessy, James (1959) *Queen Mary*, London: Unwin Hyman.

Rowson Davis, Janet (1990) 'Ballet on British Television 1946-1947: Starting Again', *Dance Chronicle*, 13, no.2, pp. 103-153.

Rowson Davis, Janet (1992) 'Ballet on British Television 1948-1949, Part I: Company Debuts, Teleballets, Recitals', *Dance Chronicle*, 15, no.1, pp. 1-39; 'Ballet on British Television 1948-1949, Part II: Grand Ballet Season and the French Connection, 1948-1955', *Dance Chronicle*, 15, no.2, pp. 153-190.

Rowson Davis, Janet (1993) 'Ballet on British Television 1948-1949, Part III: Ballet for Beginners, and Felicity Gray's Television Ballets', *Dance Chronicle*, 16, no.2, pp.197-247.

Rowson Davis, Janet (1993) 'Beauties on television – 1933-1952', *The Dancing Times*, November, pp. 153, 155, 157.

Rowson Davies, Janet (1995) 'BBC Swan Lakes', *The Dancing Times*, June, pp.877-883.

Rowson Davis, Janet (1996) 'Ballet on British Television: Christian Simpson, Producer, 1949-1959 – Divine or Diabolic?', *Dance Chronicle*, 19, no.1, pp. 17-92.

Sheean, Vincent (1956) *Oscar Hammerstein I: The Life and Exploits of an Impresario*, New York: Simon and Shuster.

Sissons, Michael and Philip French eds. (1963) *The Age of Austerity 1945-1951*, London: Hodder and Stoughton.

Sorley Walker, Kathrine (2006) *Cyril Beaumont: Dance Writer and Publisher*, Alton: Dance Books.

Turner, Barry (2011) *Beacon for Change: how the 1951 Festival of Britain helped to shape a new age*, London: Aurum.

Van Damm, Vivian (1952) *Tonight and Every Night*, London: Stanley Paula and Co.

Williamson, Audrey (1948) *Ballet Renaissance*, London: Golden Gallery Press.

Williamson, Bill (1990) *The Temper of the Times: British Society since World War II*, Oxford: Basil Blackwell.

INDEX

Royalty are listed by first names: Elizabeth, George, etc.
Bold numbers indicate page number of a related illustration.

CPSIA information can be obtained at www.ICGtesting.com
Printed in the USA
LVOW08s2143080114

368611LV00007B/1066/P